Disease

D I S

E A S E

IN SEARCH OF REMEDY

Peter M. Marcuse

University of Illinois Press
Urbana and Chicago

Library of Congress Cataloging-in-Publication Data

Marcuse, Peter M., 1914–
    Disease : in search of remedy / Peter M. Marcuse.
        p.   cm.
    Includes bibliographical references and index.
    ISBN 0-252-02215-7 (cloth : alk. paper)
    1. Medicine—Philosophy. 2. Medicine—History. I. Title.
R130.M346   1996
610'.1—dc20   95-19707
                                                              CIP

To my family—
Hazel, Yvonne, Dan, Jeanne, and Jo

Contents

Preface

Since time immemorial humans have tried to understand the nature of disease and to obtain relief from suffering. For many centuries these attempts involved fantasy or superstitions, such as the belief that demons, vicious animals, or unfavorable stars cause illness. The eighteenth century saw the beginning of rational explanations and ushered in a period of rapid progress.

Medicine can rightly be proud of what physicians and other scientists have achieved. Most people, including many outside the medical profession, are nevertheless aware of the unexplored territory that still lies ahead. We have come to realize that many of the tasks we believed to be solved are still with us. New threats from environmental pollutants, viruses, and bacteria resistant to antibiotics are but a few of the many reasons for sobering thoughts.

Our knowledge of the causes behind specific morbid conditions is fragmentary. We have been slow to learn that there is often a principal cause that must be associated with a variety of secondary factors before it becomes effective. Most important in this causative network is the genome (genetic makeup), which determines whether a particular person will be vulnerable to the principal cause of a disease. Finally, we are gradually coming to understand the role of risk factors that enter the causative complex and may remain undetected for long periods of time. Such risk factors include erratic changes in the environment and fluctuations in our physical condition.

In this book I attempt to do justice to the accomplishments of medicine without losing sight of its shortcomings. This reservation implies that we must exercise caution in our demands and expectations. We see human beings trying to be "in phase" with the environment. The attempt fails when we unknowingly introduce risk factors inherent in new technology and in drugs that we had regarded as beneficial.

We cannot expect to promote our health without using judgment and restraint in our personal life-styles. Without applying the proper limits on our expectations, we will make excessive demands on the medical profession. This "gimme" attitude leads to an enormous financial responsibility for the government, which it must pass on to us all.

Disease has plagued men, women, and children of each generation. Will human genius ever succeed in completely understanding the nature of this scourge? It is elusive and changes its strategy unexpectedly. At the end of the second millennium we have no master key to the enigma.

In the search for a solution, qualified authorities must examine any research results over adequate periods of time. Without this precaution it is impossible to prove conclusively whether the drug has a beneficial effect—or severe delayed side reactions.

Promising reports in the news media that are not related to drugs also warrant caution instead of uncritical acceptance. Some newspapers and magazines are already talking of future large-scale victory by gene engineering and are hinting at the extension of the human life span to 200 years or more. These visions may be based on occasional statements by scientists but are not likely to materialize, at least not in the foreseeable future.

No law may dictate to us that we cannot dream. When we awaken, however, we must face reality and see medical progress as a road without an end. The land that is free of all ailments is Utopia, cloud-cuckoo-land. *Homo sapiens* should not expect it now, in the next millennium, or beyond. The enigma of disease will remain, and with it remains the challenge to make steady progress in the fight against the elusive phantom.

■

My gratitude is due, first of all, to my wife, Hazel, without whose untiring efforts and encouragement this book could never have been completed; to my friend and colleague Dr. Herbert L. Fred, who was always ready to assist me with his experience and helpful advice; and to the administrative and editorial staffs of the University of Illinois Press, who were most cooperative, knowledgeable, and a pleasure to work with.

My heartfelt thanks go to all of them.

1

Into the Void

And the earth was without form, and void;
and darkness was upon the face of the deep.

—Genesis 1:2

Into the void has come life. The static calm gives way to its throbbing, glittering vitality. In the archaic wilderness there is the beginning of a purpose, of ordered motion and development.

The brink of life. The creatures are molecules, a few atoms from the primeval slime, linked to each other and molded into functioning structures. Their function is mere existence for a minute moment. While they live, they act seemingly as separate units, capable of independent action and physically disengaged from their environment. This sovereign existence is deceptive, however, for each creature is only an extension of the vast mass of matter from which it has sprung. Its atoms quickly dissociate from one another unless they maintain an interchange with the original pool.

Time, a seemingly endless passage of time. Myriads of living molecules prove to be failures, unable to establish lines of successive generations. Still, the thread of life persists in those beings that have overcome all adversities. In the course of eons the survivors become more complex in their structures and functions. Molecule is added onto molecule, and organic compounds are joined together.

The cell emerges as the result of a long and tedious experiment of nature. This unit is immensely well suited to cope with its environment, to adjust to unfavorable conditions and to synthesize its own food from the elements of air, soil, and water. Its status as a subordinate component of the outside world is the same as that of the first animated molecule. The cell must interact smoothly with its surroundings, or it will die. It receives sustenance from the environment. It must transform these products to render them suitable for its own metabolism, and it may succumb to any substance that it cannot force into a compatible form.

Time. Huge lapses of time, seemingly empty, yet full of subtle metamorphosis. The unfolding sequences of evolution lead to specialized monocellular organisms: bacteria, protozoa, viruses. Cells acquire nuclei. They procreate by means of sexual reproduction. Cell is then added to cell, and life enters a higher level of organization represented by plants and animals.

The task of coping with the outside world has now become more difficult for each being. No longer is its dependence confined to the inorganic pool around it; now it must also deal successfully with other beings. Animals may eat plants or other animals. Bacteria can invade or destroy the tissues of animals, while the white blood cells of the victim, in turn, could kill the invaders.

The force of life now has proliferated to populate the earth with creatures of every size, shape, and color. The maintenance of life is no longer an all-or-nothing proposition. Each highly developed organism has built-in devices that compensate for adverse influences. Failure to cope with the environment need not be fatal but may cause a state of malfunction and declining vitality. This condition is reversible, but unless terminated by adjustment or repair, it will eventually be fatal. Initially it is only a deviation, hardly noticeable at first, yet potentially painful, crippling, and lethal. It is a gray zone, belonging to life yet slanted toward death.

More evolution. Much more refinement in the organization of plants and animals. Mutation and selection are nature's principal tools. Certain minute changes in the genetic code prove important in the course of time and favor survival of a species. After the fishes, the reptiles, and the amphibians come the mammals. Above all, there is the development of the brain in some species, culminating in a variety of apes, superapes, sub-humans, and at last, *Homo sapiens*.

The human body, regardless of its highly developed build and function, is still subject to the basic law of nature. It cannot divorce itself from its environment. Its tissues must receive nourishment and oxygen from the outside; the blood in its veins needs water and must be maintained at a suitable temperature. Even if these fundamental needs are met, death may still come from the environment in the form of other living creatures, poisons, radiation, or one of many other inanimate objects.

Whereas animals and plants respond to environmental influences with stereotypical reactions, humans make decisions that are the product of their educations, experiences, and individual judgments. Furthermore, humans evaluate the environmental situations by means of stored knowledge.

These distinguishing attributes of humankind mean an unceasing effort to explore and improve. They lead to an awareness of the good and the bad. Whatever is pleasant or useful to us we call good, and everything that brings pain or sorrow we call bad. We learn to associate the gray zone of life with pain, disability, and impending death, an evil that is of the greatest concern to us.

Living among the plants, animals, and inanimate objects, we have learned to observe, record, and correlate. Like the other animals, we are aware of any loss of vitality within ourselves, but we also analyze this feeling and try to explain it. The dimming of vitality causes a state of uneasy existence linked with distress and anxiety. It is the opposite to the ease of our normal day-to-day living. It is *disease*.

In the imaginations of people in traditional cultures, this invisible tormentor and killer is a sinister force, most powerful and greatly to be feared. A single spirit might personify the cause of all suffering, or a host of demons could be responsible, each inflicting a specific ill by physical means. In the words of a Vedic hymn from about 1000 B.C., "When thou, being cold, and then again deliriously hot, accompanied by cough, didst cause the sufferer to shake, then, O, Fever, thy missiles were terrible."[1] This simple concept knows only two physical states, health and disease. Health is normal, good, the friend of humankind. Disease is deviate, evil, and destructive. The evil spirits invade the body, and only the magic of the shaman can drive them out.

The critical human mind does not long remain satisfied with this naïve view of illness and health. Through the centuries questions are asked and better answers sought. Students listen to their teachers, first in the shadows of trees or in crude huts and later within the peristyles of temples, the colonnades of monasteries, and finally, the amphitheaters of universities.

At first superstition and childish imagination furnish an easy solution to the problem. Disease, the wizards say, befalls humankind in the form of a feared animal. The wolf tears the skin, leaving raw flesh. The serpent's bite makes sores or blisters, and the crab tortures its victim by pinching and gnawing. Medical terminology perpetuates this primitive belief: lupus (wolf), herpes (serpent), cancer (crab). In this worldview animals are supernatural beings to be feared and revered. Their goodwill must be bought with gifts of food. An amulet of wolf's teeth or a girdle of wolf hide will keep disease away. Eating parts of a sacred animal or drinking its blood has healing power.

Slowly the human mind gropes toward rational explanations. Disease is seen as the effect of a specific, physical cause. The bad air in the swamps brings malaria. This is the beginning of realistic conclusions that lead to the discovery that mosquitoes carry and transmit the causative microorganisms (*Plasmodia*) of malaria.

Progress suddenly accelerates. Many ailments are attributed to microbes and effective remedies discovered. The cause-and-effect principle helps scientists to unmask obscure conditions and find cures for them.

But controlled research also leads to new problems. The cause-and-effect relation is complicated by hitherto unconceived factors. Highly virulent microbes, for instance, may be harmless to persons who have immune antibodies against them. Under some circumstances, however, antibodies can themselves be harmful. They may bring death to the infants of Rh-negative mothers, and there are even conditions in which a person's antibodies are believed to attack his or her own tissues.

Near the end of the twentieth century we know that disease is surely not a demon or a wild animal seeking to destroy us. Neither is it simply a microbe coming from the air to enter our lungs, make us sick, and kill us. Humanity, it seems, has to start fresh—if not from the beginning—in dealing with disease. The cause-and-effect principle is still valid, but the task of relating the cause to the effect has become infinitely more complex.

The scientist of the twentieth century is aware that health and disease are biological states, reflecting the body's smooth or faulty contact with the environment. Anticipation of the body's reaction with any possible environmental contact might lead to the avoidance or modification of all hazardous contacts. This would mean prevention of disease, the ultimate goal of health care. Scientists must also realize, however, that they have yet to find a clear, all-embracing definition of the nature of disease. They know only that it results from an interplay of forces and that the effect is enhanced, weakened, or nullified by prevailing conditions.

The entrance of microbes into the body is opposed by immune antibodies, white blood cells, and local tissue resistance. It is favored by low temperature, poor nutrition, and injury. The strength, weakness, or absence of any factor will introduce variations, and this accounts for the large number of possible conditions that decide whether the microbes succeed.

Already more than six factors are known to govern bacterial infections, and still more are bound to be discovered in the coming decades. The laws of mathematics postulate a staggering number of variations, depending on fleeting changes within the body or the environment. Still, with the aid of a steadily improving technology, we expect to cope with astronomical figures.

Could a computer accurately calculate the likelihood of disease from the combination of all influential factors? The potential formula would have to be sufficiently flexible to accommodate any new factors that research might bring to light. In the twentieth century the rapid progress of the science of genetics has uncovered additional determinants of disease. What had been called a person's constitution or genetic makeup has been analyzed and defined, and partial answers to some ancient questions have been found.

Among these questions are the following central ones: Why are some families predisposed to certain ailments? Why may disease be present at birth? The answers were traced to traits that are inherited in a predictable manner. Subsequent investigations determined the sites and mechanisms of genetic control. Geneticists recognized that the traits reside in genes, which occupy fixed locations on the chromosomes within the nuclei of the cells. Painstaking research eventually identified deoxyribonucleic acid (DNA) as the "stuff of life," representing the genetic code, which is the pattern for all physical properties of the body.

Nonetheless, the geneticists' exploits have not diminished the role of the environment as a determinant of disease. On the contrary, the outer world has taken on greater importance, for it has been shown to alter organisms' genetic properties. Genes are known to undergo mutations through exposure to radiation, chemicals, or viruses, and general external conditions like heat and cold may cause mutations as well. The emergence of genetics has made the concept of health and disease more complex, because it introduces notions not only of inherited properties but also of the possibility of mutations.

Near the end of the second millennium A.D., humans cannot expect a computer to calculate their health at any given time. The ideal solution would be an equation expressing disease (d) as the difference between all disease-promoting (p) and disease-opposing (o) combinations, assuming that the former is greater than the latter.

$$d = p - o$$

It is safe to predict that humankind's knowledge of p and o will grow steadily but will always remain fragmentary. The true nature of disease, like the essence of life and death, will forever be shrouded in mystery. The equation is destined to remain an ideal. The knowledge of its quantities can be approached but never fully attained.

■

Billions of years after it first came into the void, life on earth is still subject to up-and-down fluctuations. Its quality is seldom, if ever, without flaw, and disease thrives in its shadow. We have ventured into outer space, set foot on the moon, and sent probes to the planets. We have learned nothing, so far, that points to the existence of any extraterrestrial life. Nonetheless, when we look at the sky on a clear night, we often wonder whether there might not be living creatures on the planets or on a planet circling one of those millions of faraway stars in other solar systems. What might that life be like? Primitive or highly developed? Perhaps those distant beings, if they do exist, have attained the utopian state that we on earth can probably never reach: life free of famine and war, and above all, free of disease.

2

The Unit and the Whole

The significance of the constituent parts will
at all times be found only in the Whole.

—Rudolf Virchow, "Cellular Pathology,"
in *Disease, Life and Man*

"**W**hat does disease mean?" asks the
child. The father answers, "It is something that makes us sick." He sees
the child's blank expression and wonders what it *does* mean. He tries to
explain further: "Something goes wrong with us."

"How do we know it has gone wrong?"

"We know because we don't feel right." The father begins to realize that
he cannot explain what may be wrong before he knows what is right. Right
for every man, woman, and child, for every animal and plant. Right for
any being, whether it consists of just one cell or many million, as long as
it is a living unit.

From early childhood we are trained to think in terms of units that we
tend to regard as self-contained entities. A person is a unit, and so is a
microbe. How could each be anything but a being separate from all other beings and all things? Is not each body enclosed in an envelope of skin
that clearly marks its boundaries? We seldom stop to think of the continuity between the constituents of the body and what is outside it. The air

in our lungs is a direct extension of the atmospheric air. All body fluids, as well as their chemical contents, are fractions of the external stores of water, minerals, and organic compounds. A portion of our bodily contents can at any time be safely assumed to have belonged to the land, water, or air around us only a second earlier. The space bounded by the skin is not sealed off from the vast space around it. On the contrary, the chemical constituents of both flow into each other and become inseparable.

When we realize this continuity, we see the body as a temporary localization of matter borrowed from the pool within which it exists. This existence continues only as long as there is sustained exchange of additional matter with the pool. Survival thus depends on uninterrupted communication with the bulk of matter of which each being is a part. Apparent units are only subdivisions, not independent entities.

If we are now asked to name the "whole" to which the fractions belong, we are at a loss for a precise definition. To be sure, they are parts of the living population residing on earth, but they also have contact with inanimate matter and depend on an uninterrupted supply of it. Their need, moreover, exceeds terrestrial confines and includes a requirement for the radiant energy of the sun, as well as possibly for other forms of radiation from outer space. Our definition, therefore, will lack precision, since we can say only that all biological units are divisions of cosmic matter and energy.

Rudolf Virchow laid the foundation of modern pathology while he taught at the University of Berlin during the second half of the nineteenth century. One of his great contributions was the identification of the cell as the fundamental living unit. "Life," wrote Virchow, "is cell activity. Its uniqueness is the uniqueness of the cell."[1]

A biological unit may be a single cell, without a nucleus and showing hardly any signs of organization, or it may be a complex organism composed of millions of cells. Regardless of what constitutes the unit, whether it is minute or large, simple or intricate in structure, it is inseparable from its connections with the whole, the mysterious entity that defies exact identification and that we can describe only as the total of all forms of matter, living and inanimate.

In this jungle of creatures and lifeless objects, each biological unit must maintain an uninterrupted communication and exchange with the whole to survive. It lives in community with other units that compete with it for food, air, water, and other necessities and that, furthermore, may attack it as predators. There is a grim likeness between the primitive biological community and civilized human society, where fellow citizens are competitors and where nations attack one another with deadly weapons.

An individual unit can survive only if it maintains communication with the outside. The necessity for this interrelation was recognized by the great pioneer in physiology Claude Bernard, who taught in Paris during the mid-1800s. He used the terms *milieu intérieur* and *milieu extérieur* to refer to an organism's internal constituents and the external conditions on which the organism depends. The term *milieu* is usually translated as "environment." The *milieu extérieur* comprises what we generally regard as environmental factors, such as air, water, and so on. The *milieu intérieur* is formed by the liquid part of the blood and is diffused through the tissues, which depend on its nutrition, supply of oxygen, and discharge of waste products.

Life, according to Bernard's concept, is a conflict between the two milieux. "Life is perceived only through the conflict of the physico-chemical properties of the *milieu extérieur* and the vital properties of the organism, reacting with one another."[2] The physiologist Walter Cannon later popularized the use of the term *homeostasis* to indicate a state of stability pertaining to body functions.[3] The concepts of Bernard and Cannon are crucial to our understanding of the regulatory mechanisms that control the interaction of the body with its environment. Nonetheless, these theories were still narrow in scope. Bernard thought mainly of the circulating organic liquid that surrounds and bathes all of the anatomical elements of the tissues. Cannon had in mind the balance of physiological functions through a system of internal controls.

Further discoveries introduced new ideas concerning the regulatory mechanisms of the body. The central nervous system and the endocrine glands were recognized as the principal means for maintaining optimal conditions within the organism. Nervous impulses regulate the action of organs, tissues, and cells. Hormones, the products of the endocrine glands, mediate responses to changing requirements.

The advent of genetics has added another facet to our concept of health and disease. We know now that all components of the biological unit are the products of its genetic material. In their remarkable book *Genetic Prophecy: Beyond the Double Helix*, Harsanyi and Hutton give their definition of health as the balanced interaction of the genes with the environment.[4]

But the unit's communication with the whole does not depend simply on its genes. It is subject, among other factors, to the state of its physiological functions, such as digestion and blood pressure. The effects of stress and, at least in humans, of emotions also determine how it will react with the world around it.

The unit's condition is therefore subject to constant changes. The composition of the environment, likewise, undergoes fluctuations that may be natural or artificial. The interplay between the unit and the whole is consequently marked by instability, being conducive to health at one time and to disease at another. In its attempt to maintain an equilibrium, the body uses a number of regulatory mechanisms.

Autoregulation is active at all levels of our internal structure. It governs the action of the heart, the lungs, and all other organs; it safeguards the sound condition of the tissues; and it ensures the viability of the cells and their "subcellular" components. These concepts, although still incomplete, nevertheless point the way to our knowledge of those functions that help biological units to survive in a vast array of competing beings, hostile creatures, and inanimate objects.

To stay alive a unit must not only communicate with the whole but also be in a state of perfect response with it. Water available on the outside is of no value to the unit unless the unit has the proper equipment to absorb it, store it, and distribute it to the unit's sites of need. The unit needs specific receptors for each substance that it obtains from the whole. Moreover, whatever it returns—carbon dioxide, waste products, or energy derived from the oxidation of nutritives—requires specific transmitting devices. The give-and-take between the unit and the outside is operative only as long as it is balanced. Deficient transmission or reception by the unit will destroy it. There is no conventional expression available to classify this state of perfect response, but I will borrow a term from physics and speak of being "in phase."

An organism is in phase if it meets the following requirements:

1. an adequate intake of all bodily needs, balanced by a commensurate output of energy and waste products;
2. adaptation to environmental changes;
3. protection, through avoidance or active defense against environmental factors to which adaptation is not possible; and
4. repair of damage sustained through contact with environmental factors.

The means by which the biological unit fulfills these demands varies with the degree of its organization. The amoeba can meet the intake-output requirements through primitive reactions. It engulfs its food by flowing around it, and it depends on osmosis for the exchange of water and chemical constituents. The higher animals and humans possess complex physical equipment that is capable of keeping their bodies in phase.

The regulation of intake and output is subject to the principles of Bernard and Cannon. The internal and external environments interact constantly and exchange vital matter. Homeostasis is mainly the function of the endocrine system, which is regulated by feedback mechanisms. An elevation of the blood-sugar level, for instance, will cause release of insulin, which lowers the concentration of sugar in the blood; any depression of the level inhibits the release of this hormone through a negative feedback. The chemical constituents of the blood and tissues are thereby kept within a narrow range, and deficits or excesses are minimized through appropriate exchanges with the external milieu. Stabilizing actions, pertaining to a multitude of physiological states, occur simultaneously and incessantly, each designed to keep the biological unit attuned to the vast outside. If conditions on the outside are static, this complex mechanism should guarantee that the organism will remain in phase with the whole. Under these circumstances the biological unit would be in its ideal state, which implies a life of serenity and permanent well-being.

Nature is not geared to static quietude, however, and the environment of each unit changes constantly. Atmospheric conditions and the availability of water, food, and shelter are erratic, and any organism lacking the ability to adjust to these variations will soon perish. Furthermore, living beings are faced with the unpredictable emergence of alarming or threatening situations. A rumbling sound might indicate danger from a falling rock. An approaching animal may have hostile intentions. Human beings associate many sounds and sights with implications of danger, and their bodies make appropriate adjustments even when danger is not actually impending.

The work of Hans Selye, which has brought him worldwide acclaim, gives us an insight into our adaptive functions.[5] According to Selye, stress is the body's nonspecific response to any demand made on it. The various stress-producing factors, called stressors, each elicit essentially the same stress response. Prolonged exposure to cold has much the same biological effect as an extended period of pain.

Selye postulated further that any exposure to a stressor leads to an increase in the performance of body functions, with the ultimate aim of restoring balance. Each organism, however, has definite limits beyond which it can no longer withstand the effect of the stressor. The initial alarm reaction leads first to a stage of resistance, and resistance yields to the stage of exhaustion if the stress persists. This triphasic reaction characterizes the general adaptation syndrome theorized by Selye.

Again, the physiological manifestations of the syndrome are identical for different stressors. The primary manifestation is a stimulation of the adrenal glands, which secrete hormones and thus effect changes in the types of white blood cells present and in the blood's chemical constituents. These changes include an elevation of the glucose level, which makes more glucose available to the muscles for a rapid defense action after the initial alarm. The sustained general alarm syndrome, when observed in animal experiments, causes shrinkage of the lymphatic organs, ulcers of the stomach and intestines, loss of weight, and changes in the chemical composition of the tissues and body fluids.

The results of the animal experiments suggest a close connection between stress, adaptation, and disease. Selye summarizes this relation as follows: "There is an element of adaptation in every disease; but, in some maladies, the direct effects of the disease-producers, in others the body's own defensive adaptive reactions, are more prominent. Only in the latter case do we commonly speak of *diseases of adaptation.* Usually adaptation consists of a balanced blend of defense and submission. Some diseases are due to an excess of defensive, others to an overabundance of submissive bodily reactions."[6] The concept of stress in humans has become associated with harmful emotional effects that are held responsible for diseases of adaptation, such as peptic ulcers, high blood pressure, and some forms of heart disease. This application of the stress theory is still subject to controversy, but the principles of adaptation and the alarm reaction are well established.

Alarm signals, most of them minor, flash almost without letup in the daily life of any human, for there are always changes taking place in the environmental conditions. Most of these evoke automatic adjustments of body functions, for instance, contraction of the pupils in response to strong light. In these instances the alarm fulfills its function of keeping the body attuned to the outside. The ongoing adjustment of the body's internal system is the means by which it adapts to the environment. "Adaptability," says Selye, "is probably the most distinctive characteristic of life."[7]

The nature of the environmental change, however, may be so severe that the body cannot adjust. In that event the alarm will be the signal for escape or defense. The arm brushing against a hot stove is retracted through reflex motion. The escape has been accomplished, but the original balance is not completely restored. A small burned area of the skin remains, ready to form a blister. The mobilization of local defenses begins before the break of the blister can give bacteria access to the damaged tissue. The blood vessels increase in caliber, thereby delivering more blood to the burn site, and with the blood come leukocytes, which are special antibacterial weapons. This is the first stage of inflammation, a defensive process that, although painful, signifies resistance to invasion. After the blister breaks, microbes enter through the opening. The dead tissue would be an ideal medium on which they could thrive, but they succumb to the action of the leukocytes and other bactericidal agents that are activated by the inflammation. The final stage begins with the sloughing of the dead tissue and ends in the closure of the gap through the regrowth of connective tissue and epidermis.

A review of this episode in the life of a biological unit shows how intricate a process is required to protect the body from relatively minor adversities. The sequence of events began when an external force threatened to upset the balanced state of the organism by an excessive elevation of its temperature. The instant alarm reaction involved coordination of the nervous system with the muscles of the arm, resulting in escape with minimal damage. A second alarm signal came from the burned skin and initiated the tissue's defense against bacterial invasion. Closure of the hole in the skin completed the operation, which by combining escape, defense, and repair kept the organism safe from external damage.

Ordinary phenomena of nature evoke in us a feeling of mystery that tends to become more profound when we try to explain them. To look at the starlit sky is an ever-new romantic experience. When we begin to realize the vastness of the sparkling display, however, with distances so great that some stars have burned out before their light reaches the earth, our look at the sky becomes more than a familiar experience.

Similarly, our view of the many forms of life is tinged with shades of the fantastic when we let our thoughts penetrate into their states of existence. We know that every being is a unit composed of innumerable subunits, each of which fits snugly in its place and performs its tasks fluidly in cooperation with the other components. The composite structure is tuned perfectly to function as a unit, with internal devices guaranteeing coordination of the different parts.

In spite of their flawless construction, however, the individual creatures cannot exist in a vacuum. Their *milieu intérieur,* so vital to their inner balance, would become degraded and soon be lost if it were not in a constant state of interchange with the external environment. We might think of the living organisms as being suspended in this exterior. It acts as their nutrient, supplying them with their required solid, liquid, and gaseous matter. Unless all these needs are met, death must result from dehydration, starvation, or suffocation.

When we become aware of the necessity for constant adjustments, retreats, attacks, and mending operations, we begin to understand the magnitude of the task and its intricacies. If the unit is to survive, it must remain in phase with the whole. Even without any interference from external changes, there is an ongoing revision of the internal milieu, since the intake and output of vital substances are variable.

A single facet of physiologic chemistry, the maintenance of blood pH, illustrates the complexity of this task, because it entails a number of processes that must run simultaneously. A smooth reproduction of this technique in industry would tax the ingenuity of the best chemical engineer. The pH, which is a measure of hydrogen concentration, indicates acidity or alkalinity. The human body maintains a blood pH of approximately 7.4, signifying a slightly alkaline state. To keep this pH stable the blood must have in it a buffer system that can minimize shifts in either direction. There must be excretion of carbon dioxide by the lungs and of fixed acids by the kidneys. Finally, phosphoric acid must be removed from the blood by way of the intestine.

The stabilization of pH is only one phase in the control of the blood's chemical equilibrium, and this in turn is but one of many balances that the body must hold. Constant changes in the requirements for energy are met by the production of adrenalin and other hormones. This system is vital when an emergency calls for an immediate state of readiness. In that event the action of the hormones provides more blood sugar, which the muscles can quickly convert into energy. There is also a sudden rise in the pulse rate and blood pressure so that a larger volume of blood will reach the muscles and other sites of action. The response of the body to the ever-changing conditions of the environment constitutes a clockwork of unimaginable complexity. On it hangs the existence of the biological unit, side by side with other units, each being a part of an unknown total.

What is right? Being in phase with the whole is right for the unit, and the unit will prosper as long as it remains perfectly attuned to the outside. The maintenance of this balanced state requires more precision than the theories of Bernard and Cannon, ingenious as they are, can explain. Nonetheless, our limited knowledge is sufficient to make us see how much can go wrong with what has to be right if we are to live.

Even if all the regulatory devices function perfectly, the balance of the internal system may be abruptly destroyed by the intrusion of viruses, bacteria, or other foreign substances, so the body relies on sophisticated safeguards against this hazard. Inflammation is one of the fundamental forms of such defense. The migration of leukocytes to the endangered area and the associated rush of blood account for the cardinal signs of inflammation, which are redness, swelling, heat, and pain. We can see in this disturbance the essence of the body's defense mechanism and its relation to disease. When bacteria invade the skin, the external environment has transgressed on the internal system and threatens to destroy it. There is a throbbing pain, and the victim is aware of being sick, but this distress stems from the body's effort to overcome the infection and restore its internal balance. The relation of pain to the defense against invasion is the key to an understanding of any illness. Disease is the indicator of damage to the internal system caused by the environment.

Inflammation represents a model of prompt and effective response to an external challenge. It embodies some strategic principles that are keynotes of modern warfare. The invasion is detected without delay, and mobilization of the defense is initiated automatically. The supply line of the invaded territory is utilized to the greatest extent possible. Most important of all these features is the mechanism that guides the defenders to the target, since the invaders activate specific substances within the leukocytes or other disease-fighting cells of the body.

An example of this mode of action is the release of *interferon* by a cell that has been infected with a virus. Interferon is a protein that "interferes" with any subsequent infection of the cell by a second virus. Interferon has attracted the interest of researchers because of its possible effect in combating cancer. An interferon-producing gene can be spliced into the DNA of microbes, and the precious substance is then harvested in relatively large quantities.

The leukocytic reaction, with all its spectacular built-in devices, is still simple when we compare it with the more comprehensive system of immunity that provides a specific response for each external challenge. It is a system designed to discriminate between "self" and "nonself" and to render harmless anything that is foreign to the organism. Sir Macfarlane Burnet, who received the Nobel Prize for his contribution to immunology, characterized the immune principle with the following words: "It is a self-evident fact that a man or any other vertebrate in health lives at ease with his own components, but if cellular or macromolecular material from almost any other individual is introduced into his tissues, antibody production or some other immunologic reaction is evoked."[8]

Such alien substances are called antigens and often are microbes or viruses. An immune response may be directed also against chemical agents, however, including drugs and any foreign protein. The intensity of the reaction depends on a combination of factors, particularly the nature of the antigen and the number of previous exposures.

The basic significance of immunity is easy to understand: an organism has built-in sensors that enable it to recognize foreign matter and to respond defensively. This ability is under genetic control and reflects the general principle that keeps each biological unit on guard against a potentially hostile environment.

Immunity is a powerful device that, together with inflammation, protects the integrity of the body's internal system. The functions of this mechanism are so intricate and so diverse that no human-made equipment can be even remotely compared with it. To approach the perfection of the immune response, we would have to invent a robot with the following specifications:

- It makes contact with any invading foreign matter and learns through this contact to recognize the same material at the next encounter.
- It retains the memory of any contact over a long period of time, often indefinitely.
- The functioning parts of the mechanism are stored conveniently and can be mobilized quickly when needed.
- If necessary, the reaction can be increased in strength through repeated contacts with the same stimulant.

It is unlikely that we will ever create anything that equals the immune system. We can support it with drugs or stimulate it through vaccination, and we may suppress it to retard the rejection of a transplanted heart or kidney, but we cannot duplicate its perfection.

This magic performance is an attribute of any natural defensive mechanism. When we realize this excellence of our protective devices, it is only reasonable that we wonder why they should ever fail. Since the safety of our internal system is guarded so carefully, we might expect it to be impregnable. How can there be room for disease when its emergence signifies that the internal system has come to harm? The implications of this discrepancy exceed the domain of biology and become a matter of personal conviction, for the real question is whether life is intended to follow an easy path or displays an up-and-down movement beset with periods of suffering.

Natural history gives us no more than partial insight into the conditions that account for the vulnerability of the internal system. Each cell of an organism can exist only in conjunction with other cells, and the entire organism depends on the external environment. The dependence of any unit on the whole means competition with others. It is this biological rivalry that forces the individual units to take risks.

Humankind has surpassed all other living creatures through our ability to plan, invent, and organize. In spite of this advantage, our need to compete not only has persisted but has become more compelling. The contest with our fellow humans is a cause of stress and poses a permanent threat to our tranquility, and although technology gives us more material goods, it also creates new environmental hazards. The competence of a biological unit is put to the test whenever it faces a new risk. Failure to meet the challenge means friction instead of smooth interplay with the outside world.

Nature, the great Sphinx that speaks in riddles, presents us with an apparent paradox. That disease, the antilife, can exist at all is mysterious, since nature seems so intent on perpetuating life. We may have to revise our concept of disease. Perhaps it is not really antilife but merely a biological state signaling that life is in danger and that we must protect it by adjusting our relationship to the external environment.

A unit is in perfect balance with the whole until it is confronted with a risk that it cannot surmount. The ensuing disturbance is the result of a less-than-perfect response. As long as there is competition, there will be risks and biological failures. The fact that progress inevitably leads to new risks is significant to the utopian nature of my equation $d = p - o$. We might make o (the disease opponents) sufficiently large to equal p (the disease promoters). This would reduce d (the disease) to zero. In reality, however, o means new medication or surgery, and these advances entail risks that increase p. We find in the end that d refuses to become zero, regardless of all progress.

We have reason to believe that humankind will gradually come closer to surmounting all biological failures. To attain and perpetuate the ideal state, however, would require complete harmony between the unit and the whole, and this harmony is incompatible with the essence of life.

There is an intriguing contradiction in our relation to the vast expanse that surrounds us. Our inner system is geared to conservative regularity. The keynote is the maintenance of its genetically determined structure, but it can perform this maintenance only through an uninterrupted communication with the outside. The outer environment represents the opposite of conservatism. Since it is a composite of innumerable units, both living and inanimate, it is subject to constant motion and change. In relating to its environment, the individual must cope with the unpredictable variations that surround it. A temperature of minus 10 degrees may be tolerable to an organism until strong air currents create a severe chill factor. Combined with a certain wind velocity, therefore, a minus 10 degree temperature becomes incompatible with life for this organism.

Since the days of Claude Bernard, science has developed his concept of the two milieux far beyond its original scope. The fine tuning of the internal system has yielded many of its secrets, and with that yielding has come an awareness of the numerous subtle ways by which we cope with the hazards of existence. *Homo sapiens,* being the most highly evolved of all the species, enjoys a considerable degree of independence in its relation to the outside world. Still, humans are not self-sufficient, and like any other biological unit, we can never detach ourselves from the whole.

The relationship between humans and their environment proves resistant to any attempt at a logical analysis. It resembles the condition of a vassal who is given a generous amount of freedom by his sovereign but always remains subservient to him. Modern thinking goes beyond the comfortable idea of the internal milieu as a fortress that safeguards the body against external perils. By paying more attention to the role of the environment, we realize how vulnerable we are in spite of biofeedback and other automatic reactions that are expected to guarantee our internal equilibrium. Environmental factors may break through the body's defenses and initiate a state of disease by damaging the internal system.

Of particular concern today is our own contribution to the hazards that we face. We modify the environment in ways that are uniquely human. Animals cope with natural risks by taking flight, seeking shelter, or pursuing some other instinctive action. Humans try to outwit nature by using their ability to think. We burn wood, coal, or oil to resist the cold. We gain a tremendous advantage over other creatures by making our own synthetic compounds, harnessing the elements, and splitting the atom.

New technology brings new risks, however. It introduces pollutants and other risk factors, such as radiation, into the environment. Moreover, there is usually a lag period before we become aware of the new hazards that we ourselves have unleashed.

Risks with which we cannot cope become causes of disease. In addition to the natural risks, there is now a host of artificially produced ones, and we are consequently subject to diseases of our own making. Will human beings eventually learn to live without making new risks? Past experience indicates that this is unlikely. We cannot keep from creating new ways of living, and by perfecting them we unwittingly incur new risks.

In his evolutionary theory Herbert Spencer said, "the penultimate stage of equilibration in the organic world . . . must be one implying the highest state of humanity." Nevertheless, he warns us that "scientific progress . . . can never arrive at anything like perfection."[9]

If we base our expectations on experience and probability, we see no end to the conflict between ourselves and the environment. There will be steady progress made toward a harmonious state, leading to approximation without completion. Only in the cloud-land of imagination is there a permanent equilibrium between the unit and the whole.

3

The Risks of Living

It is only by risking our persons from one hour
to another that we live at all.

—William James, *The Will to Believe*

The dictionary defines *risk* as the chance of injury or a hazard. When we say that we accept a risk, however, we imply that we expect a benefit with a reasonable degree of probability. The mathematician can express this connection in a precise formula: $r = q(e)$, where r is the risk, e is the immediate effort that should be made in the hope of obtaining a certain benefit, and q is the probability that this effort will be made in vain. For those who do not like mathematics, it might suffice to say that nothing worth having is without risk—or still more simply, that living is risking.

The human contribution to resistance against disease is not confined to the discovery of new drugs and surgical methods. The quest for a disease-free state entails much more than a search for spectacular advances, for it is complicated by the constant emergence of new hazards that are the products or by-products of technological achievements in all fields of endeavor. These substances have unknown effects that may be capable of causing disease.

Medicine itself is a prime area in which formidable dangers to our health are inadvertently created. The iatrogenic* diseases are typical representatives of ill effects that were not anticipated in the course of progress. Analgesics, antibiotics, and many other commonly used drugs can cause irreparable damage to vital organs or interfere with the formation of blood cells. Remedies that are well tolerated by most recipients will induce severe sensitivity reactions in some patients, who may become jaundiced, develop a fever, or break out in hives. Victims of these side effects will readily agree with the shrewd wit of the ancient Roman author Publius Syrus, who said that "there are some remedies worse than the disease." Drug-induced injury to the offspring may cause birth defects, as in the case of thalidomide. We have even learned from the complications caused by giving stilbesterol that this effect can be delayed for years (see chap. 5).

Health hazards of a nonmedical nature often are related to industry and agriculture. Atmospheric pollution has only recently been recognized as an obvious problem, as have DDT and other insecticides. Any improvement has its price, which cannot be paid in money alone.

Acceptance of health hazards began with the use of coal, causing irritation of the lungs and skin from coal dust and soot. Then came mechanical devices that brought stressful noise and potential injuries. We now have commercial products that may produce allergic reactions or aplastic anemia for some consumers. We also face the runoff of toxic chemicals that poison our rivers, lakes, and oceans. New compounds enter the market before they have been thoroughly tested, posing unknown threats. Moreover, even if the risks from chemical substances can be controlled, there is still the problem of disposal of nuclear wastes and of radioactive leakage from nuclear plants.

The most serious aspect of occupational exposure to health hazards is the increased risk of cancer. It was first documented in 1775 by Percivall Pott, in a report on cancer of the scrotum, which he found to be prevalent in chimney sweeps. "The disease in these people seemed to derive its origin from a lodgment of soot in the rugae (creases) of the scrotum."[1]

Coal tar was found to be the component of soot that is carcinogenic to the skin. In 1914 Yamagiwa and Ichikawa produced cancer on a rabbit's ear by painting it with tar.[2] Cook and Kennaway identified the carcinogen more specifically by isolating benzo(a)pyrene, a polycyclic hydrocarbon, from coal tar.[3]

Iatrogenic—from Greek, *iatros,* a physician—means "caused by a physician."

Subsequent observations on occupationally induced cancer included studies on cancer of the skin in persons handling arsenic. Many hazardous substances employed in industry have been identified in the past few decades. Among these are vinyl chloride and asbestos, both of which can be shown to be carcinogenic in animals. Vinyl chloride is a hazard to workers in the organic chemical industry and in the manufacture of rubber. It is responsible for angiosarcoma of the liver, a tumor that is rarely present in unexposed persons. Animal experimentation suggested the hazards of occupational exposure to vinyl chloride, and epidemiologists later confirmed them. Inhalation of asbestos fibers has been incriminated as predisposing individuals to certain tumors of the lung and possibly to malignant conditions of other organs also.[4]

It is immaterial whether the industrial carcinogens cause cancer by themselves or play only an intermediate role in its causation. The fact that they increase the risk is sufficient to be of the greatest importance to all those involved. The involvement is not confined to public health officials but extends to industrial executives, the workers, and the general public.

Recognizing the hidden dangers to our health and dealing with them efficiently may be a bigger task than finding cures for known ailments. While advancing the human-made phase of the fight against disease, we are also expanding the exposure to human-made hazards, and the technology serving their detection is primitive compared to the methods of practical medicine.

Protecting the public against hazardous substances is left mainly to government agencies that are held responsible if an approved product causes serious damage in any number of persons. To forestall damage to human beings, legislation governing approval of such substances generally has required that evidence from animal experiments be taken into account. The Delaney clause of the Food, Drug, and Cosmetic Act prohibits the "use of any substance in any amount whatever, which, when fed to man or animals, induces cancer." Indeed, we would have an easy way out of our predicament if we could identify all hazardous substances by experiments on rats or guinea pigs. But is there always a reliable correlation between the effect of a product on animals and its action in human beings?

This problem came into focus when the artificial sweeteners cyclamate and saccharin were banned by the Food and Drug Administration. The ban was prompted by experiments in which rats developed cancer of the urinary bladder after having been fed either of the sweeteners over a prolonged period of time. The Delaney clause forced the government agency to prohibit the use first of cyclamate and later of saccharin. The use of saccharin, however, was eventually authorized again.[5]

Most medical experts believed that the carcinogenic risk to human beings could not be assessed accurately from studies on animals. The differences in the amounts consumed by people and the relatively high dosage given to the rats made the implications of the experiment appear particularly doubtful. The Advisory Group on Cyclamates concluded in its report to the secretary of health, education, and welfare that "the significance of these experiments and what relevance, if any, they have to man cannot be evaluated with present knowledge."[6]

In spite of their limitations, animal tests—also referred to as bioassays—still constitute our best tool for the detection of carcinogens. Virtually all substances known to cause cancer in humans are carcinogenic in animals. Whether this statement also holds true in reverse is questionable and extremely difficult to investigate. We cannot say that all agents capable of producing cancer in animals will do so in human beings.

Our search for hazardous products has not yet been reduced to a neat laboratory procedure with precise measurements yielding conclusive information. Methods based on tissue culture are aimed at the malignant transformation of individual cells by cancer-causing substances. This in-vitro technique promises to be simpler and faster than the bioassay, but it has not been developed to perfection.[7] A practical and totally reliable in-vitro test would be an invaluable contribution to health care. Any new risk factor could be tested for its carcinogenic potential and appropriate steps taken if harmful effects were detected. It is impossible to establish the number of lives that such a test might save, but it would surely be significant.

While we are waiting for a better method, we must take the results of animal tests seriously. With the welfare of millions of exposed persons at stake, we cannot afford to ignore the opinion of experts such as Dr. Umberto Saffiotti from the National Cancer Institute, who claims that "the only prudent course of action at the present state of our knowledge is to assume that chemicals which are carcinogenic in animals could also be so in man, although the direct demonstration in man is lacking."[8]

The alternative to experimental evidence is epidemiology, which is concerned with patterns of distribution of diseases and relies on data collected from field studies. These are directed primarily at the possible ill effects of substances to which people have been exposed. The field studies make use of vital statistics, hospital records, and direct information from workers in industry, public health officials, and others. Rates of incidence and mortality are correlated with time, geographic distribution, and characteristics of individuals. The jigsaw puzzle gradually yields a descriptive profile of a disease that guides the investigators in their search for risks. If they succeed in this pursuit, they will prove that a certain factor, or multiple factors, can be linked to the profile of the disease and hence must be responsible for it. The epidemiological approach, which uses clinical experience as the acid test, is slow, and the warning bell does not sound until the health hazard has claimed victims. These painstaking efforts are nevertheless indispensable to preventive medicine. Their results have contributed greatly to the detection of lethal risk factors and subsequent reductions in the mortality related to these risks. The gradual unmasking of cigarettes as promoters of cancer, emphysema, and heart disease is an example of this tedious hunt for potential killers.

Sometimes evidence derived from clinical experience is strong but not overwhelming and thus becomes the center of controversy. This particular problem is illustrated by the side effects that have been attributed to the use of estrogenic hormones. Estrogens are products of the ovaries and are greatly reduced in quantity after menopause. The reduction often causes undesirable conditions such as "hot flashes," wrinkled skin, and brittle bones. Medication with estrogens minimizes these complications of menopause, and this treatment is therefore widely used.

A relatively high incidence of a specific cancer of the uterus (endometrial carcinoma) in women who were taking estrogens or who retained a high postmenopausal estrogenic level without medication had been observed for some time before controlled studies were initiated. The ensuing investigations confirmed the assumption that a strong association exists between replacement estrogens and endometrial cancer. Among the factors that increase the risk for endometrial cancer are the following: relatively late age at menopause; prolonged medication with replacement estrogens after menopause; and obesity. The role of obesity is explained by a physiological process that takes place after menopause, when estrogen is derived from *androstenedione,* a product of the adrenal gland. This conversion has been shown to occur at a much higher rate in obese women than in appropriate controls.

Scientific analysis of any apparent association between a risk and a disease must be critical and is often lengthy and tedious. First of all, the analysis must determine whether the observed correlation is significant or merely incidental. In the case of estrogens, critics have said that long-term use of these hormones does not cause cancer but that endometrial carcinoma is more readily diagnosed in women taking this medication because the majority of them are under continued medical observation. This argument implies that endometrial cancer often remains unrecognized unless it is specifically suspected and sought.

The evidence for estrogens being a cancer-causing agent appears firmly established, but the critical argument against it is a typical example of the obstacles to any investigation of health risks. Most observed facts admit at least two mutually contradictory explanations. A plausible rebuttal can usually be found for any claim.[9]

The problem of separating substances that are useful and innocuous from those that are also useful but have ill effects is common to the medical profession, as well as to industry and agriculture. It affects virtually all objects with which we come in contact. Because of the rapid progress of technology, there is an incessant emergence of new products that make our lives easier or more pleasant while potentially posing a risk to our health.

Each step in the development of an industry may create lethal by-products. Their effect can be slow and remain unnoticed while vast numbers of workers are exposed. Cancer-promoting factors with delayed action have been termed "cancer time bombs" and may set the stage for malignancy to appear twenty or thirty years in the future. Asbestos is an example of an industrial cancer time bomb. In everyday life exposure to sunlight is a carcinogen with delayed action that causes skin cancer in susceptible persons. Such cancers are usually slow growing and can be treated by simple excision but may sometimes be widespread and aggressive.

The time-bomb factors are not by themselves responsible for cancer, but they constitute ingredients in the carcinogenic mixture. This mixture consists of genes and other agents that have not yet been firmly established but that probably include hormones and possibly viruses. Recognition of the long-acting causes is of special importance, because individuals may be able to avoid cancer by discontinuing exposure to any of them even after it has lasted for some time.[10] An American Cancer Society directive (November 9, 1979) declares, "A program of hunting for cancer time-bombs in the environment marks a turning point for our thinking."

To plan for preventive measures is essential to any new engineering design. Methods for treating radioactive wastes so that they can be reduced to a harmless state in a short period of time have been promised but not perfected. The rapid progress of technology is a challenge to chemists, physicists, and engineers, who must build automatic safeguards into each new design. By converting one chemical compound into another, we tamper with the physical forces of our environment.[11] If we suffer damage to our bodies in this process by liberating toxic substances against which we have no protection, we are as careless as the man who is slain by a tree that he himself has felled.

Surveys aimed at the detection of factors conducive to cancer began in the early 1920s and provided models for the fundamental methods of later surveys. The pioneer researchers recognized that variations in the habits of cancer patients can be studied only with the use of controls. They found possible connections between heavy smoking and cancer, and they also suggested a hereditary predisposition to the disease. Most important, they realized that the figures of their studies were insufficient for significant conclusions, and they urged that large-scale investigations be conducted.

One of these projects was the 1941 study by two famous surgeons, Alton Ochsner and Michael DeBakey, which focused on the role of smoking in the causation of lung cancer.[12] Their observations correlated the increased incidence of this cancer over a period of eighteen years with the increase in the consumption of cigarettes during the same period. Ochsner and DeBakey concluded from this evidence that the increase was due largely to smoking, particularly the greater consumption of cigarettes.

Research programs aimed at the detection of environmental risk factors characteristically extend over long periods of time. Their results may remain questionable for years after completion of the program, and benefits often fail to materialize. In 1959 Dr. E. Cuyler Hammond and the American Cancer Society initiated "the largest human biological study ever undertaken of life and death."[13] Sixty-eight thousand volunteer workers obtained answers from 1,078,894 adults regarding the effect of lifestyle, habits, and environment on health and longevity. This enormous effort was rewarded by the identification of the following vital facts:

1. Cigarette smoking greatly increased the risk of death from heart disease, lung cancer, and several other cancers.
2. Women who were 40 percent overweight had a higher rate of cancer of the uterus and ovaries and somewhat higher rates of cancer of the breast and gall bladder. Men 40 percent or more overweight had higher risks of cancer of the colon, rectum, and prostate.

3. Death rates from coronary heart disease and stroke were far higher among men having no exercise habits than among those with slight, moderate, or heavy exercise.

Among the fifteen leading causes of death in the United States, there are three that exceed all others in magnitude. The mortality tables of 1986 list diseases of the heart as responsible for 36.4 percent of total deaths; malignant neoplasms accounted for 22.3 percent, and cerebrovascular diseases for 7.1 percent.* The situation is actually somewhat simpler, for arteriosclerosis is directly responsible for most diseases of the heart and also for cerebrovascular diseases. Malignant neoplasms, furthermore, represent conditions that are generally called cancer. In its widest sense, this term pertains to all malignant tumors of specific tissues or organs and also to malignant conditions of the blood-forming tissues, including leukemia.

In short, arteriosclerosis and cancer are the foremost killers, and their control represents the most urgent problem to be solved in health care. For neither of these two conditions can we define a specific principal cause, but we do have known risk factors for each. The detection and subsequent verification of these risks is crucial, for their elimination will reduce the number of deaths from these two diseases.

Research into risks for arteriosclerosis and cancer is limited because of the tedious nature of the available methods. The bioassay is in many ways helpful in the study of cancer, but very little of this approach is applicable to the investigation of heart disease. Clinical observations, and particularly epidemiological studies, have been necessary to determine what factors might be conducive to the degenerative conditions of the blood vessels.

Many of these investigations concern diet, which, aside from genetics, appears to be the principal factor in arteriosclerosis and an important factor in cancer. To study dietary habits, as well as other aspects of lifestyle, it is helpful to examine population groups that are either at a relatively low or high risk for these two diseases. The high-risk groups are often occupational, for example, workers in industries that expose them to certain carcinogens. Low risk is indicated by a low incidence and a relatively low mortality compared to that of the general population.

Certain religious groups observe prescribed life-styles that regulate

*Vital Statistics of the United States, 1986.

their diets and many of their nondietary habits. When the incidence and mortality statistics of cancer and heart disease in these groups are compared with those outside the groups, significant differences are observed. The Seventh-Day Adventists, for example, abstain from alcohol, tea, and coffee. Most members do not smoke and follow a diet that is low in meat and fish. A few are complete vegetarians. The church has recommended these dietary habits for over one hundred years. Life-style is further regulated by an emphasis on religious teachings, self-discipline, and the importance of the family.

Comparative studies have correlated the health status of members of this denomination with that of control groups. The results indicate that Seventh-Day Adventist men have a lower incidence of coronary disease, as well as a low incidence of cancer of the lung, bladder, mouth, larynx, and esophagus. In women the mortality from postmenopausal cancer of the breast, ovaries, and uterus was below that of the general mortality figures. The incidence of cancer of the cervix was also lower. For both sexes the risk of death from cancer of the colon, stomach, and pancreas was about 70 percent that of the general population. Blood-pressure readings in the vegetarian members were significantly lower than in the nonvegetarian controls.

Other religious groups with strictly regulated diets and habits also rank above the average population in matters of health. Members of the Church of Jesus Christ of Latter-day Saints (Mormons) abstain from tobacco, alcohol, tea, and coffee. They do not abstain from meat but observe moderation in its use and recommend a balanced and regular diet. The incidence of cancer in this group is low, as is the mortality from diseases attributable to arteriosclerosis. The cancer death rate of whites in Utah, where there is a large Mormon following, is about 75 percent that found in the total white population of the United States.[14]

The difficulty in drawing conclusions from studies of religious groups lies in the large number of risk factors that their teaching excludes and habits that they advocate. The general rules usually stress conservative social practices. It is not possible to identify any specific cause of cancer or heart disease by comparing religious denominations with other population groups, but these studies are nevertheless of great value. They show that risks can be minimized by simple rules governing our personal conduct in many spheres of life and that control of life-style may be expected to bring health benefits.

Some projects have been designed so as to allow researchers to pinpoint individual risk factors in a population group over a period of years. The Framingham Project has followed a population sample in the town of Framingham, Massachusetts, since 1948.[15] Its main purpose is the detection of risk factors underlying cardiovascular disease. This category includes coronary heart disease, heart failure, cerebrovascular disease (strokes), and peripheral vascular disease (arterial disease involving the extremities). Project participants must be free from all these ailments at the start of the observation.

Repeated examinations make detailed data available for each member of the group. This information includes cholesterol levels, lipoproteins of high and low density, blood pressure, size of the heart, and possible evidence of diabetes. Using this information, the project's researchers designated different risk categories and determined the incidence of coronary heart disease for each category. It has been apparent that the occurrence of coronary heart disease in an individual can be predicted fairly accurately from that person's risk category. The chances of developing a cardiovascular disease by age sixty-five were 37 percent for a man and 18 percent for a woman in this study.

In the first twenty years of the Framingham Project, about 6 percent of the women and 8 percent of the men were diagnosed as diabetics. Incidence of cardiovascular disease in diabetic men was twice that of nondiabetic men; for women, it was three times higher in diabetics than in nondiabetics. Diabetes thus constitutes a definite risk factor for cardiovascular disease.

Large-scale projects are necessary if we want to be aware of risks to our well-being. Through such studies we gradually come to see some of these hazards as being particularly serious. Measures must be taken to forestall the effects of these hazards, which come in many forms. Occupational risks consist mainly of exposure to carcinogenic chemicals, and employers are usually responsible for protecting the workers from them. Health authorities are expected to protect the populace from pollution of air or water by toxic chemicals and from radiation. This leaves a large number of risks whose management is the personal responsibility of the individual and that can be termed voluntary.

The existence of voluntary risks is important as a reminder and a warning. We cannot ensure a perfect state of health, yet neither can we deny that neglect and abuse favor disease. As advances in science detect more causes and devise new preventions for our ills, the individual obligation becomes increasingly important.

Risks that are voluntary and avoidable can be found almost anywhere if one looks closely. By accepting the meaning of responsibility in its broadest sense, we come to suspect that all our ills are someone's fault. Many are the result of our own life-style. Some could have been foreseen and prevented by generations before us, and many are related to neglectful practices of industries or communities. In the most general way, society and all humankind stand accused of having been slow to provide solutions to our health problems, and each of us must share in the blame.

This kind of reasoning recognizes the importance of personal choice in relation to one's health and logically leads to a demand for enforcement of health rules by a system of rewards and penalties. It is not surprising to hear suggestions that premium rates for health and life insurance should be geared to a person's risk status. A bona fide nonsmoker deserves a better rate than a smoker. A man with high blood pressure could have his rate increased for failure to obtain adequate medical attention during the year. Conversely, there might be a bonus for regular medical examinations and screening procedures, such as the determination of blood pressure and blood sugar, as well as Papanicolaou smears.

As justified as this system might seem, there is a need for restraint in any attempt to sell it to the public. The problem lies mainly in the predictive power of the individual risks. Deciding whether a voluntary risk—for instance, lack of regular exercise—is really responsible for more illness and a shorter life span requires years of controlled studies by medical investigators, statisticians, and actuaries. There are sources of error that can hardly be controlled—the type and amount of exercise; the person's state of health before the start of the program, diet during the program, and liability to mental strain; the climate; and many other variables.

Individualized calculation of risks is the basis for counseling on health preservation. A computer can furnish a life-expectancy score based on an individual's personal data. These data include (among other things) occupation, habits, family health, height, weight, blood pressure, and blood cholesterol level. A woman may have a score indicating that her life expectancy is ten years less than average unless she makes certain adjustments, such as giving up cigarettes.

The recognition of risk categories is necessary in medical practice, even if they are only probable rather than definite. Physicians are under an obligation to adjust plans for the treatment and observation of their patients according to potential risk factors. A woman with a high incidence of breast cancer in her family needs frequent examinations of her breasts. An obese man who has a desk job should have less food and more exercise than a laborer of normal weight. These are strictly medical considerations, intended for the benefit of the individual. "We are not yet sure," the doctor might explain, "that you are at high risk, but I cannot afford to take any chances with your health and must advise you accordingly."

To inject these complicated and often controversial considerations into public life is a matter quite different from their medical applications. Bureaucracy would seize this opportunity to assign people to categories, to keep records of their risks and make special rules for them. Men and women would find themselves penalized for failure to avoid certain risks that research later might prove to be irrelevant. By that time the memory banks of the computers in the business offices and governmental agencies already would have stored the information on the poor risks, and it would never disappear from the victims' records.

Personal life-style, habits, and diet are important to our health. Each of these factors is subject to our control and is therefore our responsibility. This means that we have to make decisions according to our own judgment instead of simply following printed regulations. Individual choice enters into all fields of life except where freedom has been lost entirely. There are no hard-and-fast rules that might be applicable to everyone. Saving money regularly brings prosperity to some, while others fare better by risking their revenue on speculations.

Where our health is concerned, we look to the medical profession and the public health agencies for guidelines. We must always remember that their advice is at best based on results of research and that different information might come at any time. To follow bookishly every word of advice that is spoken or printed makes us turn into pathetic figures, so busy holding onto life that we have little time to enjoy it.

There are no guaranteed results in any endeavor, health care being no exception, and few pieces of today's knowledge are immune to revision by tomorrow's evidence. Official enforcement of health rules would necessarily take its cue from many kinds of research, including animal experiments, clinical investigations, and statistical data. Much of this information will be controversial, however, and some even conjectural. Once the bureaucratic machinery is set in motion, it cannot stop, wait, and examine but must continue to function. Letters would go out to millions of citizens:

Dear Sir or Madam,
You have been assigned to Risk Category 25A, due to your continued use of salt, sweeteners, and certain fatty acids, as well as your lack of morning exercise and irregular sleep schedule. Accordingly, you are assessed additional penalties for which you will be billed separately.

Had such a system of compulsory regulations been put into effect in 1970, it would have been credited with the remarkable improvement of health statistics that took place during the following decade. The report of the secretary of health, education, and welfare made in 1980 notes a large decrease in the death rate of the past ten years for males and females in all groups. The number of deaths caused by heart disease declined 17 percent. Infant mortality dropped from 2 percent to 1.4 percent. Life expectancy at birth increased by 2.3 years, from 70.9 to 73.2 years. Since citizens' private health care was not regulated by law during the 1970s, we may assume that the improvement was due to advances in the medical field, voluntary health measures practiced by individuals, and public health control of pollution and other risks.

Except for enforcement of public health rules, there was no penalty system in the 1970s. Would the statistics have been even better if we had lived with penalty points? We do not know, but we had best be satisfied with the present achievement and not ask for more regimentation. Anyone who is familiar with government safety regulations for business and industry knows that these lists have grown longer year by year and that some of the rules simply cannot be obeyed in practice. If a similar system applying to personal health care were enforced, many of us would be chronic offenders and simply accept our penalties.

Individual health care requires personal initiative. It cannot be delegated to an "Office for the Prevention of Voluntary Health Risks" or any other agency. The causes of the principal killer diseases, cancer and arteriosclerosis, are still under investigation, but there is good evidence that they are somehow related to our life-style, particularly our smoking habits, diet, and exercise.

In each walk of life we come to a point where we must make a choice. A lawyer may advise us on intricate legal matters and then say, "The decision is up to you." Doctors can try to detect disease and treat it by the most advanced methods. They will tell us that it is best not to let disease establish itself, but they cannot give us a simple, guaranteed guide to prevention.

When we are in unexplored territory, we often must rely on common sense and sometimes relinquish the desire for absolute safety. In the thicket of health rules it is impossible to discriminate between truth, half-truth, and misinformation. On all sides we are confronted with alarming advice on diet, exercise, and environmental hazards. If we want a completely guided tour through life and try to heed all warnings, we become neurotics living on a starvation diet.

Disease indicates the individual's failure to cope with risks and to compete with the rest of the biological world. Pneumonia is a victory for bacteria or viruses; diabetes is a metabolic defect that an individual must overcome if he or she wants to live.

Our best weapon in this ongoing battle is our ability to think, which includes making personal decisions on matters of health. To take reasonable risks is as necessary as taking precautions. We choose to risk as long as we do not feel that the nature of the hazard has been convincingly established. We heed warnings that are based on reliable studies by qualified experts, but we ignore suggestions voiced by alarmists who accept circumstantial evidence without critical examination.[16]

A computer may assign us to a risk category, but the computer's verdict is subject to individual judgment. Each person is responsible to him- or herself. Science gives us information resulting from current research, but if we wish to benefit from up-to-date evidence, we cannot wait for iron-clad confirmation.

The principle of acceptance or rejection applies to each of us in health matters, just as it holds true in business, politics, and other spheres of life. Our wrong choices are our *own* choices, and we must accept responsibility for the consequences, be they poverty, war, or disease.

The very meaning of choosing implies a degree of uncertainty. Without this element of doubt all selection would be automatic and not subject to intelligent decisions. The physical state of animals is entirely dependent on automatic functions. Humans add to this self-regulatory mechanism their ability to act independently according to personal choice. They must accept certain risks in shaping their state of health. General George Patton's wartime record qualifies him as an expert on the subject of risks. His advice, given in a letter to his son, Cadet George S. Patton IV, holds true not only for military operations but also for peaceful endeavors. He wrote, "Take calculated risks. That is quite different from being rash."[17]

The Causal Connection

Insofar as the causal connection is thought
about merely by means of the intellect, it is
a nexus constituting a series of causes and
effects that is invariably progressive.

—Immanuel Kant, *Critique of Judgment*

When the apple hit the ground, Isaac
Newton related its fall to the gravitational pull of the earth. The effect had
been linked to its cause, and the cause-and-effect principle had prevailed.
The rigid concept of "A follows B" is a crucial law of the exact sciences. It
performs almost without exception in their territory, but it has limitations
when applied to biology. Not that biological events are exempt from the
laws of physics, but they are often so complex that a single cause cannot
account for them adequately.

In medical discourse a condition is frequently identified as the "cause"
of another condition. Hardening of the arteries is said to cause heart disease. This explanation is unsatisfactory, however, unless we know what
is responsible for hardening of the arteries. For some ailments there is a
more meaningful explanation. Tuberculosis is caused by infection with
the tubercle bacillus. This is a plausible and rational explanation, but why
do some persons contract this disease while others do not? Why does one

victim have a mild form of tuberculosis and another is gravely ill? We will be less confused and disappointed if we approach our search for the causes of disease more cautiously. We might think of a system with the biological unit in the center and the environmental forces around it. As long as the unit maintains a flawless performance within the system, disease fails to materialize. Tuberculosis, for instance, may not pose a serious threat, provided that

a. the body's immune mechanism is intact,
b. nutrition is good,
c. external temperature is within normal range,
d. lung tissues are not damaged by irritating smoke or toxic fumes,
e. circulation of the blood through the lungs is unimpaired,
f. the right ions are exchanged at the right time,
g. hormones and enzymes are released in proper amounts, and
h. physiological reactions still unknown to us safeguard the functional integrity of the organism.

After we have been introduced to this multitude of "ifs," we will no longer wish to accept only one cause for any particular disease. Each cause has its own cause(s), and individual causes compound one another. This complexity has led biologists to reject the mechanical theory.

John Scott Haldane, the great British physiologist, made fundamental contributions to our knowledge of respiration. When he investigated the effect of high altitudes, he moved his laboratory to Pike's Peak in Colorado. His methods of investigation followed the rigid standards of scientific tradition, yet he professed to be a "vitalist," concerned with life rather than any mechanical force. "As a physiologist," wrote Haldane, "I can see no use for the hypothesis that life, as a whole, is a mechanical process. This theory does not help me in my work; and indeed I think it now hinders very seriously the progress of physiology. I should as soon go back to the mythology of our Saxon forefathers as to the mechanistic physiology."[1]

Will Durant, the renowned historian and philosopher, is even more outspoken in his condemnation of mechanistic thinking in biology. In his book *The Pleasures of Philosophy* he predicts, "And when biology is at last freed from this dead hand of the mechanistic method, it will come out of the laboratory into the world; it will begin to transform human purposes as physics changed the face of the earth; and it will bring to an end the brutal tyranny of machinery over mankind."[2]

Durant's argument, supported by the opinions of some of the foremost biologists, has its merits. Humans are not machines, and neither is any other living being. Nonetheless, what goes on inside any living organism still must obey the laws of the exact sciences; at least, we expect this absent proof to the contrary. The difference between human and machine lies in the extreme complexity of living matter and the many facets that have not yet been sufficiently comprehended.

What we call the cause of a disease is usually a risk factor that, enhanced by other factors, has disturbed the biological state. It has become a determinant of disease, and it acts in concert with other determinants to form a causal complex. One component of this complex is the principal factor, such as the microbes or viruses in the infectious diseases. The principal factor, however, asserts itself only in a suitable setting with allied factors and in the absence of effective opposition.

In the case of an infectious disease such as tuberculosis, the principal factor is the tubercle bacillus. Its ability to cause disease is favored by a host's poor nutrition and exposure to other infected persons. Immunity, the action of leukocytes, and the response of body tissues at the site of the infection all counteract the tubercle bacillus. The "for" and "against" forces are equal at one moment, and the biological state is in balance. At the next moment, however, a new factor—chilling temperature, for example—may be added to the complex and tip the scales in favor of tuberculosis. Disease takes hold when conditions are just right. It is an indicator of imbalance between the "for" and "against" forces.

This explanation of how tuberculosis starts is an extremely simplified one. In reality the various factors are much more numerous, as are their possible combinations. Occupational hazards, air pollution, and personal hygiene are some of the variables that influence susceptibility to an illness. The abundance of the "for" and "against" forces makes it virtually impossible to predict an individual's chances of contracting a specific disease. Even if we considered only a majority of variables instead of all of them, we would have to make complicated calculations. It is questionable whether a computer could be adequately programmed for that task. Mathematical precision can seldom be expected when life processes are involved.

The laws of physics can be applied against a background of known constants and variables. In biology, however, it is often impossible to anticipate or detect subtle changes that may occur at any time. The cause-and-effect relationship is clearly apparent in the fall of Newton's apple, but it is much harder to understand when applied to the causes of disease.

Persons moving from one geographical location to another experience environmental changes that introduce new factors conducive to disease. Geographical pathology, therefore, can yield important clues for the study of causal complexes. The relation of several diseases to a common environmental factor was one of many astute observations that Dr. Denis Burkitt made while working as a surgeon in Africa.[3] He pointed out that these diseases have a common pattern and are prevalent where exposure to this factor is greatest. Appendicitis, diverticulosis of the colon, and polyps and cancer of the colon have a relatively high incidence in countries where refined carbohydrates have replaced whole-grain products rich in cellulose fibers.

Absence of a certain host factor is often necessary before an environmental agent can precipitate disease. For instance, some persons lack the enzyme glucose-6-phosphate dehydrogenase. This deficiency is genetically transmitted by a sex-linked mutant gene of intermediate dominance. Persons having this defect are prone to hemolytic anemia marked by massive destruction of their red blood cells. These attacks of anemia are precipitated by an unusual sensitivity to substances that most people tolerate. Among the precipitating determinants are drugs, particularly antimalarial primaquine. These individuals are also sensitive to the fava bean, which is a common food product. They suffer from favism, a serious form of hemolytic anemia in which the enzymatic defect acts as a *permissive* condition before the bean or its products can become the *precipitating* determinant.

Deficiencies of enzymes, hormones, or other normal constituents of the body are common permissive conditions often having a regular pattern of inheritance. The inborn errors of metabolism, first described by Sir Archibald Garrod in 1909 (see chap. 5), are examples of congenital deficiencies. In the absence of a specific enzyme, an ingested substance may not be assimilated properly and will cause disease by being stored in abnormal form. Glycogen, for instance, accumulates and damages the liver and kidneys of a person lacking the enzyme glucose-6-phosphatase.

In phenylketonuria (PKU) the lack of the enzyme phenylalanine hydrolase leads to the accumulation of phenylalanine in the tissues and blood.[4] This is a recessively inherited condition that can be detected in the newborn by a screening test and treated with an appropriate diet. If left untreated, the metabolic defect may result in mental retardation (phenylpyruvic oligophrenia).

Some common diseases stem from basic defects that lead to an inability to maintain vital bodily functions. Victims of sickle-cell anemia have inherited the mutant sickle gene from both parents. The red blood cells of these individuals are sickle shaped. They contain an abnormal type of hemoglobin, their survival time is reduced, and their oxygen-carrying capacity is impaired. Various tissues of the body suffer secondary damage that predisposes them to infection and degenerative changes.

Investigation of chemical properties have shown that the difference between normal hemoglobin and sickle-cell hemoglobin consists in a change of a single amino acid in one of twenty-eight peptide fragments. Thus, one gene controls the nature of a single amino acid and thereby becomes the determinant of a disease belonging to the diseases designated "molecular" by Linus Pauling, who was twice a Nobel laureate (see chap. 5).

Sickle-cell anemia provides another intriguing facet to our knowledge of the causal complex. There is circumstantial evidence that, in areas of endemic malaria in Africa, the higher incidence of the sickle-cell gene may be the result of natural selection. This is a plausible concept, for sickle-cell hemoglobin confers relative resistance to malaria parasites, especially in children.

According to this theory the causal complex is centered on a risk, the exposure to malaria. As a response to the risk, there is a gradual increase in the frequency of the mutant gene carrying the sickling trait, which constitutes a potential determinant of sickle-cell anemia. Disease emerges from an interplay of environmental factors and host factors governed by the laws of heredity.

Lack or insufficiency of a host factor is well illustrated in diabetes mellitus,* which is characterized by inadequate production of insulin, a hormone responsible for the regulation of the blood glucose level. The beta cells of the islets of Langerhans in the pancreas are the specific site of insulin formation. A definite genetic pattern has not been established for diabetes, which nevertheless is known to run in families. The hereditary background is especially apparent in diabetes beginning in childhood, the most serious form of the disease.

Diabetes is Greek for "running through" and refers to the large amount of urine sometimes voided by these patients. *Mellitus* is Latin for "sweet"; it is used to indicate that the urine contains sugar.

The intricate ways in which diabetes damages the body have still not been explored completely, but we know that the blood vessels are severely involved and that the presence of the disease constitutes a risk factor for arteriosclerosis. Diabetes affects 2 to 4 percent of the U.S. population and is an example of an intrinsic defect (insufficiency of insulin). This deficiency is the host factor that permits an ordinarily harmless external substance (glucose) to become a determinant of disease.

A theory that still lacks confirmation postulates yet another external factor as the precipitant of diabetes. There is evidence that a virus may damage the islet cells in genetically predisposed individuals. Mumps, Coxsackie (group B, type 4), and rubella are the main viral types that have a possible connection with diabetes. We might carry the theory further and assume that an external event, such as natural radiation, was originally responsible for a gene mutation and initiated the permissive factor for diabetes. We would then have three environmental agents—radiation, virus, and glucose—entering into the causation of diabetes.

Whenever we think that we might have a complete picture of diabetes, research comes up with yet another facet, like a piece of a jigsaw puzzle that we had overlooked. Investigators have found autoimmune antibodies in the serum of diabetics. These are antibodies directed against the islet cells of the pancreas. It might be that the original virus infection damaged the beta cells, and the products of this damage stimulated the production of antibodies that remained active after the virus had disappeared. This would mean adding another host factor, antibodies, to the causative complex. Finally, obesity, the fifth host factor, may enter the complex by changing latent diabetes to the overt form.

In all probability there are many more determinants of diabetes and also many more opposing factors that protect most people against this condition. If all the agents acting for or against diabetes in a particular individual were known, the terms of the equation $d = p - o$ would assume awesome proportions.

Having seen some examples of the intricate background of disease, we begin to grasp the immensity of the nexus that Kant sees as constituting a series of causes and effects. Without pretending to bring this extremely complicated matter down to a few simple statements, I will formulate some thoughts about the causes of disease.

Causes are born of risks that the biological unit has failed to deal with adequately. The result of such a failure is a determinant of disease that must combine with other determinants before it can place the unit in jeopardy. In any causative complex there are external factors constituting environmental risks that all units must face.

It makes sense to think that any loss of our physical well-being has an external cause. We have a right to assume that humans, like any other creatures, exist as a part of an integrated system. It would be absurd to imagine the individual as an isolated unit that thrives for a while on its own and then, also on its own, develops internal defects until it finally runs down and disintegrates. That may be the case in an engine or some other mechanical device, but it is an unlikely concept for any living organism. Individuals, be they humans, animals, or plants, exist only as parts of a total entity and not as separate units. They are dependent on one another for the maintenance of their lives and also affect one another in many ways that are hostile to life. Instead of witnessing machines performing by themselves, we see live creatures interacting, each having to adjust constantly to the changing combination of forces. As long as the process of adjustment is effective, the individual is in phase with the whole and is supported by it. Failure of adjustment means that the outside effects are no longer met by proper counterbalance; they consequently become injurious, causing the individual's decline and eventual death.

The external cause is effective only if coupled with a specific defect of the internal mechanism of compensation. This claim is subject to skeptical criticism, however, for external causes have not yet been identified for all diseases. The leading causes of death still lack sufficient exploration to allow a clear view of their relations to our environment. The available knowledge, however fragmentary, points in each case to effects from the outside and dispels the notion of conditions coming about by themselves. Unopposed risk factors have eventually been identified for diseases that were originally termed "ideopathic," meaning self-originating. The concept of disease as a state of internal decline without any specific external cause is usually seen to be erroneous in the light of scientific evidence.

It is challenging to see whether the theory of the causative complex can be applied to a list of mortalities. Table 1 indicates the leading causes of death in the United States in 1990.[5] Before we turn to the leaders of the list, however, we might look at the less-common causes of death.

At first glance, many of the causes seem easy to understand, but they become more difficult when we try to explain them. Accidents, for instance, are fourth on the list. What could be simpler to explain than a fatal

Table 1. Mortality for Leading Causes of Death in the United States, 1990

Rank	Cause of Death	Number of Deaths	Death Rate per 100,000 Population	Percentage of Total Deaths
1	Heart diseases	720,058	225.8	33.5
2	Cancer	505,322	174.0	23.5
3	Cerebrovascular diseases	144,088	43.5	6.7
4	Accidents	91,983	33.6	4.3
5	Chronic obstructive lung diseases	86,679	28.1	4.0
6	Pneumonia and influenza	79,513	23.3	3.7
7	Diabetes	47,664	15.7	2.2
8	Suicide	30,906	11.2	1.4
9	Cirrhosis of the liver	25,815	9.5	1.2
10	HIV infection	25,188	8.3	1.2
11	Homicide	24,932	9.3	1.2
12	Diseases of the arteries	24,645	7.9	1.1
13	Nephritis	20,764	6.4	1.0
14	Septicemia	19,169	6.0	0.9
15	Atherosclerosis	18,047	5.1	0.8
	Other and ill-defined	283,690	94.7	13.2
	All causes	2,148,463	702.4	100.0

Source: From "Mortality for Leading Causes of Death in the United States," *Cancer Statistics 1994;* reprinted in *CA: A Cancer Journal for Clinicians* 44, no.1 (1994): 12.

mishap? Mechanical failure is self-explanatory, but few accidents are attributable to it. Most are due to human failure, such as lack of concentration, misjudgment of distances, fatigue, or recklessness.

The usual accident means inadequate performance by the victim in a situation requiring alertness and skill. The human mind has created complicated devices, but it is not always capable of using them safely. Thorough analysis of a traffic accident would reconstruct an intricate chain of events. The guilty party might have been tired or angered by a recent occurrence. His attention was perhaps distracted by the thought of coming tasks and problems. Preoccupation with what might happen in the future enhanced his fatigue after a sleepless night and made him neglect the present.

If we want to accept a collision as the cause of death—the driver's or any other person's—we must account for the human malfunctions that led to the accident. If the driver was under the influence of alcohol or other drugs, a new aspect of failure would demand explanation. Why do people turn to these toxic substances? How do they contribute to the malfunction of mind and body? We began with what seemed to be a simple cause-and-effect situation, but at the end of our analysis, we have discovered a host of contributory factors and are still faced with unanswered questions.

For most items on the list we can identify environmental factors and host factors that together form the causative complex. Pneumonia and influenza (item 6) are caused by viruses or bacteria from the environment meeting with just the right conditions in the prospective victim. We find that the "right conditions" actually include a critical setting composed of deficient immunity, hereditary susceptibility, poor circulation, exposure, and many other variables. Again, we realize that the easy explanation is not enough. There is always a maze of circumstances through which a cause finally becomes a determinant of disease, and possibly death.

Most of us are looking for concrete entities behind the mortality statistics. We want information about palpable items, perhaps harmful food or toxic fumes, viruses, or bacteria. Our minds work best when we can visualize a cause-and-effect relationship, for such a connection raises hopes of eradicating the cause and thereby erasing a line from the mortality table.

In our quest for definite causes, we think mainly of external factors in the environment. They are more easily seen as hostile elements than are congenital defects or other conditions within our own bodies. Moreover, we expect the guardians of our health to scan the environment for possible hazards and to eliminate them speedily.

This task is considerably more difficult to achieve than it is to contemplate. Looking for determinants of disease is like sifting mountains of sand in search of a few rare pebbles. When we locate a likely object, we have to ascertain that it is genuine by subjecting it to a rigid examination. Similarly, before a risk factor is linked to any specific disease, it must meet a set of strict criteria. These include, among other things, consistency of evidence, temporal sequence, and strength of association. In more informal language, this means that the same result must be obtained in study after study, the alleged cause must precede the disease, and the cause-and effect relation must be clearly evident instead of being faintly suggested. Furthermore, the epidemiological findings must be consistent with those from other research methods, such as animal experiments. The observations must have predictive capacity, meaning that they will hold true in new study projects using a different population group. Finally, the criteria include independence of associations: if a substance is said to be responsible for a variety of diseases, it must be shown to be able to cause each of them independently. The knowledge of these standards helps us to understand the problems that beset any study in epidemiology. Thoroughness is the keyword for investigators, and they have a right to demand patience from the public.

In spite of these difficulties, we can identify external causes for most of the conditions on the mortality table. Cirrhosis of the liver (item 9) is often, but not always, related to alcohol consumption, which is without doubt an external cause. Where alcohol can be reliably excluded, we may find a history of hepatitis; in that case, the hepatitis virus is the external determinant of the cirrhosis. In rare instances the disease can be caused by certain chemicals that damage the liver tissue.

There is no problem in naming external agents for the items that rank eighth and eleventh on the mortality table. Instruments of suicide and homicide are too numerous for any brief listing. Suicide has been committed by using available objects in a great many ways, from gently inducing "sleep" with barbiturates to killing oneself by repeated ax blows on the head. With regard to homicide, any medical examiner's department collects over the years a voluminous file of external death-dealing devices.

What causes the suicide victims' decision to use these instruments of death? If we could evaluate such a person early, we might discover a complex psychological background, perhaps frustrated love, business failure, or social maladjustment. Often it is an incurable illness that is itself of unexplained cause. There are almost always multiple conditions, internal or external, that enter into the causative complex of a suicide.

We can incriminate the environment for almost every category in our table. Congenital anomalies are no exception. Injuries to the mother damage the fetus, and in a more insidious way, chemicals can do the same. Even before the infant has been conceived, damage to ancestral chromosomes by radiation may set the stage for a congenital disease.

Our problems in defining causes stem from the first three tabulated categories. We find that diseases of the heart rank first, malignant neoplasms, second, and cerebrovascular diseases, third. We can simplify the first and third items by explaining that the great majority of diseases of the heart are due to coronary heart disease,* which in turn is a result of arteriosclerosis. Cerebrovascular diseases are represented mainly by strokes, which are due to arteriosclerosis also. Heart disease and cerebrovascular disease are secondary conditions, and we have to understand the process that affects the arteries if we want to improve the mortality rates in the first and third categories.

Arteriosclerosis, which now is usually referred to as atherosclerosis,† is characterized by clogging and later by hardening of the arteries. It had long been regarded as a gradual degeneration of aging blood vessels, similar to what is expected to happen in old plumbing pipes. Eventually, however, investigators raised questions. Why do young people occasionally die from coronary occlusion? Why does postmortem examination sometimes reveal arteriosclerosis in children and even in infants? What is the substance that clogs the arteries, and where does it come from?

Some of the answers came over one hundred years ago when the fatty nature of the deposits in the arteries was recognized by Rudolf Virchow, the "father of modern pathology," and then identified more specifically by Ludwig Aschoff, another German pathologist, as lipid with a high content of cholesterol.[6] In 1913 a group of Russian investigators produced deposits in the arteries of rabbits by adding cholesterol to the animals' diets. At the end of World War I Aschoff linked arteriosclerosis in humans to their intake of food. He noted that postmortem observations revealed a decline in arteriosclerosis during a period of famine or immediately thereafter.

Following these initial discoveries, more than sixty years elapsed without any definite conclusions regarding the principal determinant of arteriosclerosis. This does not mean that science stood still. On the contrary, extensive research projects on heart disease have been conducted, resulting in a great deal more knowledge about the risk factors that are condu-

---

*The coronary arteries supply the heart muscle. Obstruction of these arteries due to arteriosclerosis causes heart attacks.

†*Atherosclerosis* refers specifically to arterial disease associated with deposits of fatty substances. It is now often used in preference to *arteriosclerosis*, which is a more general expression.

cive to the disease. The main instruments of study were a number of large-scale surveys of population groups in which different risk factors could be specifically observed.

In addition to the people in the Framingham study mentioned in chapter 3, there were other groups on which the effect of diet, life-style, or drugs could be observed. Some of these projects provided for a diet low in cholesterol, whereas a control group received a regular diet. In the Helsinki study, for instance, two hospitals were used, one of which gave only low-cholesterol food to its patients. After some period of time this hospital reported a lower death rate from coronary heart disease in men* than did the control hospital, which had provided an ordinary diet for its test patients. Similar surveys were conducted in the Chicago and Los Angeles studies, but these included certain modifications. The diets in these studies regulated not only cholesterol but also saturated fat and total caloric intake. In all the projects, death and clinical evidence of coronary heart disease were significantly more frequent in the control groups.[7]

There were also studies conducted that made use of drugs such as clofibrate and niacin, which are known to lower the cholesterol level of the blood. Reduction in the cholesterol contents was associated with a lower rate of coronary heart disease. This was of theoretical importance only, however, since the safety of these drugs with regard to other diseases could not be ascertained at the end of the study.

Responsible experts have drawn very cautious conclusions from the results of the various large-scale investigations. There is fairly general agreement that a constellation of factors is associated with the occurrence of coronary heart disease. Three factors stand out among the others, for their presence increases the risk of coronary heart disease many times. The main factor is a high level of serum cholesterol. The others are elevated blood pressure and the habit of smoking cigarettes.

Many additional facets of practical value have emerged from the painstaking surveys. These are briefly the following:

- The degree of arteriosclerosis varies directly with the content of cholesterol in the diet and inversely with the content of polyunsaturated fats in the diet.
- Estrogen and thyroid hormone diminish the plasma cholesterol levels.

*The results observed in women were not significant statistically.

- Diabetes predisposes to high cholesterol levels and arteriosclerosis.
- Some persons, although not diabetic, have a congenital predisposition to high cholesterol and arteriosclerosis.
- High-density lipoproteins protect against arteriosclerosis, whereas low-density lipoproteins promote it.
- The high caloric value of fat increases the risk of overweight, which accelerates the arteriosclerotic process.

Studies of arterial disease related to diet cover particularly difficult territory, and we consequently must be prepared for setbacks and disappointments. For example, suggestive evidence indicated that lipids other than cholesterol might be the cause of arteriosclerosis. Persons with elevated levels of serum triglycerides seemed to be in a high-risk category for heart attacks. Screening of blood samples for triglycerides was therefore performed routinely, and persons with abnormal values were placed on appropriate diets. The triglyceride theory, however, did not stand up under critical scrutiny after large-scale trials. Consequently, a group of scientists has recommended that widespread screening and treatment of healthy persons for elevation of these lipids be abandoned until more persuasive evidence becomes available.

More discouraging than the reversal of a single piece of evidence is the confusion that has been fostered by the often contradictory statements from official sources. In 1979 the U.S. surgeon general urged that Americans eat less red meat, which contains more fat than white meat. He argued that individuals with diets high in saturated fats and cholesterol usually have greater risks of heart attacks than do people eating a low-fat, low-cholesterol diet. A few months later the American Council on Science and Health said that there was no firm evidence that such a diet would in itself lower the risk of coronary heart disease. It seems that government and science have made us wait a long time and given us little aid after making us pay for many long-term projects.

To the public, the confusing scientific testimony has been disheartening and tends to destroy widely held hopes for the prevention of heart disease and strokes. How do people feel on reading these sobering reports after they have been on low-cholesterol diets for years?

It is indeed confusing to receive opposing views from authoritative sources. Nevertheless, is that not what happens in all areas of life until the dust settles after years of arguments? Are the opinions of experts on economy, energy, and foreign policy less confusing? The true picture emerges later, when today's evidence is seen from the vantage point of tomorrow. Most of us want to reap the fruits of research as soon as possible. If we wait for confirmation, it might be too late to prolong our lives. This is a personal decision for each individual. If we choose to accept recent evidence, we must be prepared for disappointment.

The long-term results of changing to a diet low in animal fat and cholesterol is discouraging at first glance. Adherence to this diet over a period of years will lower the cholesterol level by only 10 to 15 percent. If this seems a small reward for a great effort, we might ask ourselves whether a low-fat, low-cholesterol diet is really a severe physical deprivation. What, we wonder, did humans eat before we devised means of making more food available through agriculture, storage, and eventually food processing?

Our bodies may not be geared to a steady, plentiful supply of food, and even a reduced diet is possibly still more than we can handle. Some persons have a hereditary ability to keep their cholesterol low regardless of their intake, but many people exceed their safe level even on a low-cholesterol regime. Intermittent starvation is closer to the natural state of human beings than regular eating is, no matter how well controlled it might be. The decline of arteriosclerosis during a famine supports this view.

Whenever we make changes in nature's blueprint, we pay for it in some manner. We sense the meaning of this law when we hear of toxic chemicals, radiation hazards, or side effects of drugs, but we seldom think of it in connection with our supply of food. Whether we recognize the implications of this particular law actually makes little difference in our long-term policies, for another law says that we do not willingly give up anything that makes life easier, stills hunger, or alleviates pain. We will find ways of minimizing arteriosclerosis, but they are not likely to include a return to intermittent starvation. The methods must be compatible with our physical comfort, or we will prefer the disease to the remedy.

Although some of the results of research may be obscure, most of them are still suitable for use as practical guidelines. People with diabetes or with a strong family history for heart disease should watch their intake of fat more closely than others need to. A relatively high proportion of low-density lipoproteins in the serum also makes a low-fat diet advisable. The fortunate ones who are not in any known risk category must still control the amount of fat in their food or it will go to fat in their bodies and make their blood vessels age prematurely.

We have learned a great deal since the days of Virchow, after all. Nobody has discovered *the* cause of arteriosclerosis. Its principal determinant remains unknown, and any simple means of preventing heart attacks is therefore yet to come. At present we nonetheless can discern some facts among all the uncertainties. The connection between fat intake and arteriosclerosis has been proven, and a few detailed features are known.

This knowledge already affects the daily habits of millions of people. Many are likely to have profited from the adjustment, particularly those in the high-risk categories. Mortality from coronary heart disease has been declining by about 2.5 percent annually since 1968. This change, one might argue, could reflect variations that are unrelated to the changes in diet or life-style. The decreased death rate could be due to better hospital treatment of patients with heart attacks. The lower number of deaths from heart attacks, however, nevertheless suggests that we are on the right track.

More important than the modest practical results of the new knowledge is its impact on our outlook. We are now entitled to a line of reasoning that is reassuring compared to the void of years gone by. Arteriosclerosis is not simply a gradual clogging of blood vessels representing an aging process over which we have no control. It is, like all diseases, an indicator that our biological performance needs adjustment. We may be eating the wrong food, exercising too little, or worrying too much. We might need hormones or vitamins that we now have available or those that might yet be discovered.

Exactly what we have to do, or what we must not do, is only partly clear; in any event, we must find the faulty link between our bodies and the outside world. Heart disease, the number-one killer, has causes that develop from risk factors. The Framingham project and other similar studies have shown that persons who are at high risk for coronary heart disease are also at high risk for strokes and the other manifestations of arteriosclerosis. This observation simplifies the search for a common cause that may account for the deaths in categories 1 and 3 of the mortality statistics.

There is likely to be not a single cause but rather a causative complex resulting from risk factors that become determinants of disease. Dr. Daniel Steinberg, professor of medicine at the Division of Metabolic Disease, University of California, states that atherosclerosis is, in fact, a disease of multiple interactive etiologies,* and prevention may well require intervention along different lines."[8]

Etiology means "the *study* of causes," but it is often used to mean "the cause."

We can rightly believe that some factors of the causative complex have already been identified and that we have begun to minimize them with some apparent benefit. Dietary cholesterol and total fat intake, smoking, overweight, lack of exercise, diabetes, and hypertension—these are the main determinants of arteriosclerosis to which research has pointed. They are no doubt not the only causes, and others are certain to be found and dealt with in the future. Many studies concentrate on the theory that injury to the endothelial coat of an artery may be crucial to the origin of arteriosclerosis. The endothelium is the normally smooth lining of the artery. It constitutes the inner surface along which the blood flows swiftly and evenly in normal circulation.

There is good evidence derived from animal experiments and human postmortem findings that damage of the lining initiates or favors penetration of serum lipids into the wall of the artery. In addition to the lipid infiltration, there may be aggregates of blood platelets or blood cells at the site of the injury. As to the cause of the damage, our information is still limited. We can only say what it *might* be. Repeated variations in blood pressure could lead to excessive stretching of the arterial wall with gradual thinning or tearing of the endothelium.

Congenital abnormal conditions, although rare, indicate that some causative factors reside in the host. Familial hypercholesterolemia is an inherited abnormality characterized by an excessive level of cholesterol in the blood serum. Its most severe form is the homozygous type, in which the individual receives the abnormal gene from each parent. Evidence of progressive coronary heart disease may develop in the offspring during childhood. In addition, postmortem studies of coronary arteries have occasionally revealed an unusually thick lining to be already present in infants. It is reasonable to assume that individuals with this abnormality are predisposed to coronary heart disease.

Congenital predisposition, although important to our understanding, is not yet amenable to medical intervention or preventive measures. The search for causes, therefore, centers on external factors that can be avoided or modified. For example, elements in the water supply have been associated with the incidence of heart disease, but this correlation has not been convincing.

An intriguing possibility has been proposed by investigators at the Cornell Medical Center. Experiments on chickens have shown that Marek's disease, a fowl disease due to herpes virus, promotes atherosclerosis in chickens. A control group of uninfected birds on high-cholesterol diets did not develop arterial lesions. The tentative conclusion from this evidence points to blood vessel damage by a virus and subsequent penetration by cholesterol. The theory is by no means applicable to humans at this time, however. If it should eventually be supported by substantial proof in humans, it would indeed be a breakthrough. We would then have a principal determinant paving the way for the individual risk factors.

We may be tempted to look beyond the day of the dramatic breakthrough and ask whether the spectacular discovery might mean that arteriosclerosis, and with it heart disease and strokes, will disappear as smallpox and scurvy have vanished. If this came to pass, we would be very close to the utopian concept of a disease-free state. More realistically, however, it is likely that the condition will remain with us even if we learn everything there is to know about its causes.

Should we advance to the stage where our knowledge is all encompassing, we would be able to postpone the onset of cardiovascular disease and lessen its impact, but we could not permanently escape the various injuries to our arteries as they occur in the course of our daily lives. The cardiovascular system, more than any other, bears the initial impact of the stress and strain of living. Sudden fright makes blood vessels contract, heightens blood pressure, and accelerates the pulse rate. Although the arterial wall is equipped for this type of strenuous exercise, it will gradually show signs of wear, and lipid substances eventually will infiltrate the wall of the blood vessel through minute defects.

What we can reasonably foresee is a slower and milder form of clogging and hardening of the arteries. The deleterious effect will be confined mainly to those individuals who have reached old age, which may mean 100 years and upward in centuries to come. They are likely to attain advanced age after decades of usefulness with freedom from heart attacks, strokes, and other circulatory ailments. Nevertheless, one or the other of these conditions is the plausible tool with which nature will, in the end, terminate each life—even if other causes of death have been subdued. Slowly and almost imperceptibly, the pipes of the vascular system become narrower and less elastic. Their capacity to convey blood declines, and with it the delivery of oxygen to all tissues is restricted. The vital life-force ebbs and comes to a halt.

We may anticipate a marked reduction of heart disease and strokes as an acceptable goal, but this kind of compromise is hardly feasible in the case of cancer. To think that in the future there will be slower-growing cancers that wait until we have reached old age does not really make sense.

Neoplastic disease is aggressive, incapacitating, and deadly. Prevention or control after early detection is the only means that promise relief. There is no scarcity of known causes linked to malignant disease. We have a large number of environmental factors, and we also know of host factors that are mainly hereditary.

The environmental factors characteristically have a long latent period during which they must act before the condition becomes apparent. One would think that time is needed to form a suitable causative complex before the malignant transformation of cells can occur. This change is not ordinarily visible by microscopic examination of the involved cells, and much of this concept is theoretical. It is probably a process on the molecular level by which components of deoxyribonucleic acid (DNA) are affected. These changes involve degradation of amino acids in the DNA molecule and possibly also substitution of one amino acid by another. The alterations influence the metabolism and growth pattern of the cell and eventually can be recognized by characteristic microscopic features. The nuclei tend to become large and deformed. Mitotic cell division speeds up, and the cells form abnormal aggregates instead of complying with the regular pattern of the tissue to which they belong.

After a variable period of time the abnormal cells proliferate at the expense of the healthy tissue, which they tend to invade and to destroy. They are able to metabolize glucose and other nutrients by a different metabolic pathway and thereby deprive the other cells of the necessary constituents. A particularly sinister aspect of most cancers is their ability to establish daughter colonies at distant sites. This occurs when malignant cells escape from the original tumor and are transported elsewhere by the blood stream or the lymphatic channels.

The sequence of events must begin with the entrance of the determinant factor into the cell or its nucleus. A great many such carcinogens are known, but their mode of action is obscure. Chemicals that are carcinogenic in humans almost always induce tumors in experimental animals, but the reverse is not necessarily true. This discrepancy pertains especially to viruses that have been shown to cause tumors in animals. The first successful experiment was performed by Dr. Peyton Rous, who in 1910 isolated a virus that causes cancer in chickens.[9] About thirty years after the discovery of the Rous sarcoma virus (RSV), its internal structure and its mode of propagation became known. It is similar to the myxo viruses, a large group of animal viruses, and it contains in its center an RNA chain combined with a number of protein units.

RSV transforms normal animal cells into cancer cells. One can witness a single RSV virus particle transform a cell in a chicken tissue culture. Many other viruses have similar properties and produce specific forms of cancer in animals. There are viruses responsible for tumors in mice, cats, birds, and other species. Leukemia in animals has been particularly related to viral infection.

The RNA tumor viruses (retroviruses) are endemic in certain animal species. They become integrated into the genes of the host cells and are transmitted from one generation to the next. Such a clear-cut relation between any virus and human cancer has not been shown to exist, but some experts in tumor research consider such a relationship to be likely and have developed appropriate theories.

In patients with AIDS, which is caused by a retrovirus, certain neoplastic diseases are frequent complications.[10] The most common among these are Kaposi's hemorrhagic sarcoma and certain types of lymphoma. In these instances, however, the AIDS virus is not likely to be the immediate cause of the tumor. Instead, the severe immunodeficiency of AIDS patients might promote the development of the neoplastic disease.

Similarly, benign or malignant tumors of the genital tract are frequently associated with the human papilloma virus (HPV).[11] The presence of the virus can be recognized by certain changes in the cells that were cast off from the cervix or other parts of the genital tract. It is still not clear whether HPV belongs to the causative complex of these tumors or only accompanies them.

The viral theory, while unproved, fits our general concept of how malignant neoplasms may start in humans. This concept is based on an interaction between carcinogenic agents and certain conditions present in the host. Many chemicals, radiant energy, and thermal energy are definitely known to cause cancer, whereas dietary components are only suspect, and proof of their causative roles is still lacking.

The carcinogenic property of ionizing radiation became known soon after the discovery of X rays when many of those persons who used the new methods without any safeguards developed skin cancers on their hands. Another indication of this phenomenon involved the painting of watch dials with luminescent material, which began around 1915. The women engaged in this work used their lips to bring the brushes to a fine point. When many of the workers died of bone cancer, it became clear that they had ingested radium or thorium, and the radioactive elements had entered their skeletal system. Modern methods of X-ray diagnosis and treatment are subject to precautions adequate to protect the patients and medical personnel.

Ionizing radiation is emitted by X-ray (Roentgen-ray) tubes, by natural radioactive substances, such as radium or thorium, and by elements that have been rendered radioactive by artificial means. Some of these radioisotopes (e.g., carbon and iodine) are useful in research and medical practice, where they are used under strict controls. Explosions of nuclear weapons and leakage from nuclear plants also liberate hazardous radioactive material.

Emissions from radioactive materials in the earth's crust and cosmic radiation from outer space constitute background radiation. This activity is a plausible cause of mutations due to chromosomal injury that might have occurred at any time in the past, long before we had X rays, radioisotopes, atomic bombs, or nuclear plants. The ultraviolet rays from the sun, although not ionizing, can still cause the development of skin cancers.

Humans are exposed to a constantly increasing number of known carcinogens. Some of these are part of nature, whereas many others are artificially produced or, more correctly, natural products modified by humans. Many new commercial chemicals are introduced each year, and an unknown number of these may later be found to have carcinogenic effects. Table 2 lists carcinogens that are of particular occupational importance. It falls far short of a complete listing, but it provides an idea of how widespread the hazard of exposure is. As the medical literature and the news media have pointed to the rising number of carcinogens, they have also reported a steady increase in deaths from cancer. Some of the increase may mean that more diseases are diagnosed correctly each year and that cancer, instead of some nebulous entity, is listed on the death certificate.

The greater diagnostic accuracy, however, can account for only a fraction of the yearly increase in deaths from malignant neoplasms. According to *Vital Statistics of the United States,* there were 162.8 deaths from cancer per 100,000 population in 1969. The rate rose to 183.9 in 1979 and to 193.3 in 1985.

Carcinogens represent risks that we incur either knowingly or inadvertently. The manufacture of asbestos-containing items is an example of an occupational risk. Without the use of strict rules and devices to protect the workers' safety, the risk is uncontrolled, and asbestos turns from a risk factor into a carcinogen. Mesothelioma of the pleura or the peritoneum,

Table 2. Carcinogenic Agents That May Be Associated with Various Occupations

Agent	Sites of Cancer	Areas Where Noted
Arsenic	Skin, lung	United States, Great Britain, Germany, France, Argentina, Taiwan, African countries
Coal tar, pitch	Skin, lung	United States, Great Britain
Petroleum	Skin, lung	United States, France, Great Britain, Austria
Shale oils	Skin	United States, Great Britain
Lignite tar and paraffin	Skin	Great Britain, France
Creosote oils	Skin	United States, Great Britain
Anthracene oils	Skin	Great Britain
Soot, carbon black	Skin	United States, Great Britain
Mustard gas	Lung	Japan
Cutting (mineral) oils	Skin, possibly respiratory and upper alimentary tract	Great Britain, Australia
Products of coal carbonization	Lung, bladder	Great Britain, United States, Japan
Sunlight	Skin	United States, Argentina, Australia, France, etc.
Chromates	Lung	United States, Great Britain, Germany, Canada
Asbestos	Lung, pleura, peritoneum, gastrointestinal tract	United States, Great Britain, Germany, Canada, South Africa, Holland, Australia, U.S.S.R., Italy, etc.
Aromatic amines, dyes, rubber	Bladder, possibly biliary tract, alivary glands	United States, Germany, Great Britain, Switzerland, et al.
X rays and radium	Skin, lung, leukemia	United States and many other areas
Nickel	Lung, nasal cavity, sinus	Great Britain, Norway, Canada

Benzol	Leukemia	United States, etc.
Isopropyl oil	Lung, larynx, nasal, sinus	United States
Radioactive chemicals	Bones, nasal, sinus	United States
Chemicals (various)	Lymphoma, pancreas	United States
Nonspecific agents		
Used in wood furniture working	Nasal cavity, sinuses	Great Britain, United States
Used in leather working	Nasal cavity, sinuses, bladder	Great Britain, United States
Soft coal mining	Stomach	United States (1 report)

Source: From *United States Department of Health, Education and Welfare: Cancer Rates and Risks,* 2d. ed. (Washington, D.C.: GPO, 1974), 71.

a relentlessly aggressive neoplasm, is specifically attributed to asbestos exposure. The same carcinogen also promotes cancer of the lung and other organs.

Anyone contemplating the role of asbestos must realize how difficult cancer prevention is. Adequate occupational precautions can be instituted only after the harmful effect of a new agent is recognized and sufficient experience points the way to effective protection. As industrial technology proceeds, more and more substances with carcinogenic properties will emerge. Many of them require fifteen to thirty years before their harmful action is noticeable.

The promise of a more optimistic view lies in the very complexity of the cancer problem. It involves more than mere contact with a causative agent. Why can some people tolerate prolonged exposure to intense sunlight, while others under the same conditions are plagued with skin cancers? We know that dark-skinned individuals are less affected by the ultraviolet rays because of their protective pigment. We know also that a rare congenital abnormality, xeroderma pigmentosum, will result in extreme risk of cancer from sunlight. The sun's rays are therefore carcinogenic agents only under certain conditions. These reside in the host, and they determine whether the carcinogen can become effective.

One of the host factors is related to age. Most malignant tumors occur in older individuals, and this age preference has been explained in several ways. One possible reason is the long period of time required for many carcinogens to produce a malignant growth. Another concept is based on the normal immunity against cancer cells, which might be lost with advancing age.

Dependence on hormones is characteristic for many tumors arising from tissues that are normally under hormonal control. Cancer of the breast is frequently dependent on estrogen, and there is a strong connection between cancer of the uterus and the amount of estrogenic hormone remaining in the body after menopause (see chap. 3). Cancer of the prostate is dependent on the male hormones (androgen and testosterone).

Hereditary conditions are particularly important host factors, for they indicate that some people are at high risk because of their family history. These persons should be screened more thoroughly than others. Hereditary cancers are often characterized by their onset at a relatively early age and by their tendency to occur at more than one site in the same person. In some instances there are benign tumors associated with or preceding the malignant neoplasm. An example of this combination is familial polyposis, in which tumors with a great tendency to become malignant occur in the large intestine. These polyps represent preclinical markers signifying the hazard to the patient. These persons must have close medical follow-up and may need preventive surgery.

Some hereditary tumors have been found to be associated with specific abnormalities of the chromosomes in more than one member of the same family. This suggests that damage to the genes may be responsible for malignancy in certain cases. Subsequent mutations change normal cells to malignant cells. Although chromosomal defects have not been identified for cancer of the breast, heredity is a recognized risk factor for this disease. Careful screening is mandatory for women with such a family history.

An environmental carcinogen is modified by other agents that may either enhance its effect or weaken it. Nutrition is one of the modifiers and accounts for the variable occurrence rate of certain cancers in different geographic locations. The high incidence of cancer of the stomach in Japan has been attributed to dietary habits, especially highly salted foods. Death rates due to cancer of the breast and cancer of the ovaries show a correlation with the per-capita consumption of dietary fats. The lower rate of cancer of the colon in the less-developed areas of the world suggests a protective effect of a higher fiber content in food.

It would be misleading to say that cancer is caused by any one type of food or that we can escape malignant disease by adhering to any special diet. The available knowledge is not sufficient to support this statement. The evidence nevertheless suggests that diet can influence the development of cancer in a positive or negative manner.

The concept of multiple causative factors helps us to explain apparent inconsistencies of neoplastic disease. Why, for instance, do not *all* cigarette smokers get cancer of the lung? The variables inherent in each person provide a partial answer to this question. We gain additional understanding from the synergistic* effect that exists between different carcinogens and puts some individuals in double jeopardy. Among asbestos workers, those who smoke have a greater chance of developing malignancy than the nonsmokers. Smoking therefore represents a cofactor with the cancer-causing asbestos.

Experts in cancer research have designed models of the causative complex. The *oncogene* theory is based on the inclusion of RNA viruses in the genetic codes of some cells.[12] A portion of each viral gene is the oncogene, which represents its cancer-causing potential. External carcinogens, such as chemicals or radiation, can "turn on" the oncogene and thereby initiate the malignant transformation of cells and tissues.

Medical history indicates that a number of different principles were successful in achieving crucial results for various diseases. Vaccination is based on a host factor. Antibiotics interfere with the action of external causes. Injections of insulin compensate for the deficiency of a naturally produced hormone. Each breakthrough meant that humankind had found a vulnerable link in the chain of events leading to disease. To think of escaping from all viruses or all virulent microbes is unrealistic, however. Similarly, it is not reasonable to think that we can avoid exposure to all carcinogens, but we may expect that they will be rendered harmless when the causative complex is disrupted.

The kaleidoscopic pattern of "for" and "against" forces and its constant variations is typical of living organisms. It distinguishes biological units from machines, which have predictable regularity. Our position in the world of biology is unique. Only we can analyze the interaction between the causes of disease and the forces acting against it. This is our most powerful weapon in the ongoing fight.

Synergism is the simultaneous action of separate forces that enhance one another. Their total effect is greater than the sum of their individual effects.

5

From Beginning to End

As soon as we are born we begin to die, and
the end depends upon the beginning.

—Manilius, *Astronomica IV*

The life of a biological unit is an incessant effort to remain adjusted to the environment. The unit performs its physiological function to obtain all vital substances and to process them according to its needs. When its contact with the environment becomes imbalanced, the unit attempts to restore harmony by adapting itself to the new conditions. Invasion by microbes, viruses, or other intruders cannot be countered by adaptation, however. The unit requires defense mechanisms for its protection against such threats.

Ideally the unit could remain in phase with the outside at all times. This state is not attainable, however, since each unit is engaged in biological competition and is in constant jeopardy from environmental risk factors. Human beings, like any other living creatures, are faced with successive states of imbalance that they must overcome to stay alive.

We might imagine the ideal condition as a straight horizontal line. In contrast to this perfect state, real life is an irregular, up-and-down movement between two horizontals. The downstrokes represent life in jeopardy of falling to the zero level, which is death. The upward movements express the body's ability to hold onto life in spite of environmental hazards.

We reach the baseline at the time of death, when all biological functions cease. By way of analogy, we wonder whether each individual's life begins at the upper horizontal level that represents the ideal state. If this were true, the organism would be in perfect balance with its environment at the moment of its conception. This analogy is attractive but does not hold up under scientific scrutiny, for the product of conception is subject to physical flaws that may terminate its life as soon as it has begun. These defects may be caused by injury to the fertilized ovum, but they can also be transmitted from one generation to the next. The blueprints for many abnormal conditions are contained in the genetic code. Heredity decrees that life, even at its onset, is remote from the ideal state.

Although humankind had known for thousands of years that certain anomalies are inherited, it long remained ignorant about the laws of inheritance. It needed almost twenty-three centuries to progress from Hippocrates' vague theory of "pangeneration" to the work of Gregor Mendel that initiated modern genetics. Hippocrates probably was speculating when he wrote, "Sperm is a product which comes from the whole body of each parent, weak sperm coming from the weak parts, and strong sperm from the strong parts."[1] Mendel reported his observations from deliberate experiments with the following conclusions: "Experimentally, therefore, the theory is confirmed that the pea hybrids form pollen and egg cells which, in their constitution, represent in equal numbers all constant forms which result from the combination of the characters united in fertilization."[2]

Since Mendel's discovery was ignored in his days, genetics had to wait for the scientists of the twentieth century to bring it to fruition. It soon became clear that the Mendelian laws were readily applicable to insects and mammals, including humans. Microscopists and biochemists provided information that correlated inheritance with certain components of the body cells. Rodlike structures within the nucleus were called chromosomes (colored bodies) because they stain deeply with some dyes. By the year 1900 biologists knew that the chromosomes of the germ cells (spermatozoa and ova) transfer the genetic characteristics to the offspring through specific entities called genes.

Each cell of the human body has forty-six chromosomes arranged in twenty-three pairs. Forty-four chromosomes (twenty-two pairs) are called autosomes. One pair constitutes the sex chromosomes and consists of two

X chromosomes in the female, whereas the male has an X and a Y chromosome. The X chromosome contains many genes representing a multitude of physical traits. The Y chromosome has very few genes, and most of these determine only maleness.

Cells divide in one of two ways. Mitosis results in the formation of new cells with forty-six chromosomes (diploid cells). Meiosis produces cells with twenty-three chromosomes (haploid cells), which are either eggs or sperm cells. Genes occupy specific locations on the chromosomes. In the case of autosomes, each gene is matched by a corresponding gene on the other chromosome of the pair, and the two genes together control a specific physical characteristic. The genes of the X chromosome are not matched by those of the Y chromosome, and the X gene exerts control by itself.

Deviations from the regular pattern of inheritance are attributed to mutant genes. Mutations are sudden jumps in the genetic sequence, and their occurrence makes an organism produce an offspring that is quite different from its antecedents. These unaccountable changes were regarded as capricious acts of nature until Hermann Muller proved that certain genetic changes could be induced by artificial means.[3] In 1927, while working at the University of Texas, he accomplished the "artificial transmutation of the gene" by treating the sperm of the *Drosophila* fly with heavy doses of X rays. This discovery, for which Muller received the Nobel Prize in 1944, established a link between inheritance and the environment, for it was an environmental agent that modified the gene structure of the cell. This experiment alone makes us realize the all-important role of the world around us by demonstrating that even inherited traits may have originated from environmental forces.

Taking their cue from the effect of X rays on chromosomes, geneticists inferred that most mutations are caused by natural radiation, which comprises cosmic rays and emissions from radioactive elements in the earth's crust. Until recently we could feel comfortable with this assumption. Natural radiation is not under our control, and we could pretend that mutations are simply an act of fate. We can no longer claim to be innocent bystanders, however, for experts on genetic intervention have estimated that mutations are often caused by artificially produced radiation or chemicals. Progress in technology therefore might mean a progressive increase in the number of mutant genes, unless we learn to control the environmental factors that are of our own making.

Over two thousand human disorders have been traced to the effect of single mutant genes. *Dominant inheritance* implies that one mutant gene is sufficient to impart an abnormal condition to the offspring. Autosomal dominant disorders are transmitted from one generation to the next by affected individuals of either sex. Each child has a 50 percent risk of inheriting the abnormal condition. Short-limbed dwarfism, a disorder of the skeletal system, is a prime example of autosomal dominance. Huntington's chorea and neurofibromatosis, both diseases of the nervous system, are transmitted in this way as well.

An abnormal *recessive* gene can express itself only if it is matched by the same abnormal gene on the other chromosome. This match, where each parent contributes identical mutant genes, is called a *homozygous* combination. In dealing with recessive genes we may encounter carriers who can pass the disorder to their offspring without having the disease themselves. A carrier is heterozygous, meaning that he or she has a normal gene combined with an abnormal recessive gene. A child of two heterozygous parents has a 25 percent risk for having the disease and a 50 percent risk of being a carrier.

Examples of autosomal recessive disorders include cystic fibrosis, sickle-cell anemia, and Tay-Sachs disease. It is probable that every individual carries a number of rare recessive genes but that these seldom cause disease since the chance for matching with the same mutant genes is extremely small. Mating between close members of the same family may increase the chances for these rare genes to be expressed. Some autosomal recessive conditions have almost exclusive incidence in ethnic or racial groups. Tay-Sachs disease occurs mainly in Ashkenazi Jews, and sickle-cell anemia occurs in the black population.

Recessive genes that are located on the X chromosome do not cause disease if matched with a normal gene on the other X chromosome. Females with a recessive mutant gene on one X chromosome and a normal gene on the other are carriers. Males have very few genes on the Y chromosome, so virtually any mutant gene on the X chromosome, whether dominant or recessive, will exert its disease-producing effect. Females therefore are rarely affected by X-linked recessive disorders. A typical example of this sort of disorder is hemophilia, which is usually limited to males. Queen Victoria of England was a famous carrier of hemophilia. The youngest of her four sons, Prince Leopold, was a hemophiliac. Two of her five daughters were hemophilia carriers, and through their daughters, who were also carriers, the disease was transmitted to the heir to the Spanish throne and to the last czarevich of Russia's Romanoff dynasty.

X-linked dominant conditions can occur in either males or females, since only one mutant gene need be present for the disease to manifest itself. This combination is limited to rare disorders, most of which involve faulty metabolic functions.

Genetic disorders are not limited to the presence of mutant genes but may involve abnormalities in the number of chromosomes or in their structure. The most common autosomal abnormality of this type is Down's syndrome (monogolism), which is characterized by mental retardation and a variety of life-threatening malformations. In most cases the genetic defect in Down's syndrome is an extra chromosome at position 21. This trisomy is caused by a chromosome pair's failure to segregate during the meiosis of the ovum or the sperm cell.

Approximately 5 percent of the children with Down's syndrome do not have typical trisomy 21; instead, they suffer from a "translocation-type" abnormality. A translocation is the transfer of chromosomal material from one position to another. A parent sometimes has a "balanced" translocation, a shift of chromosomal material without any increase in its total amount. This parent may be a carrier of Down's syndrome, and the child may have an "unbalanced translocation," which means that there is an extra dose of chromosomal substance present and that the disease will become evident.

Geneticists have succeeded in correlating congenital syndromes (sets of abnormalities) with specific errors in the chromosomes. Trisomies at chromosomes other than number 21 account for a large number of birth defects, such as cleft palate, club foot, and heart defects. Syndromes are sometimes named after their most unusual clinical feature. In the "cri-du-chat" (cat-cry) syndrome, the infant makes a peculiar catlike sound. This disorder is associated with the absence of a fragment of chromosome 5, referred to as a deletion of its short arm.

Chromosome analysis has supplied the means by which a bewildering variety of congenital conditions can be diagnosed and classified correctly. In many cases, what once seemed to be a random combination of birth defects is now recognized as a specific condition related to a characteristic chromosomal abnormality that can be viewed under the microscope and permanently recorded by photography.

The advances in genetics have already found practical applications in genetic counseling (see chap. 7). Equally important is the contribution of genetics to our basic concepts of disease. We know that individuals' phenotypes, which are their physical makeups, are the expression of their genetic heritage, called the genotype. The phenotype emerges as the product of genetic factors that are remarkably stable but nevertheless subject to the effect of outside forces. The condition of the phenotype determines how well the new organism can cope with the requirements of the environment.

When we reexamine Claude Bernard's idea of the two milieux, we find that it has been greatly enriched by the new knowledge of genetics. We have learned that the external system not only controls the organism during its lifetime but exerts a profound effect on it long in advance. The environment's prelife control of the organism is brought about through induced mutations of the genes and errors in the division of the chromosomes. In our conflict with the outside world, we face the results of events that took place many generations ago, when humans had no knowledge of genetics. The welfare of future generations will depend largely on what happens in our time. We have barely had a glimpse of the connection between ourselves and our environment, but this small knowledge imparts great responsibility.

In some instances the organism is seriously inadequate from the beginning of its existence and is doomed to almost immediate failure. In that event, the abnormality of the phenotype should be apparent soon after conception has occurred. This means that sometimes a recently fertilized ovum will be visibly deformed. During the first week following conception, the ovum passes through the oviduct into the cavity of the uterus. The mother's endocrine system makes automatic adjustments to prepare the lining of the uterus for its task of supporting and nourishing the ovum. For the duration of the pregnancy the principal hormone is progesterone, which protects the pregnancy and replaces estrogen, thereby preventing any further menstrual periods.

In about 10 percent of all pregnancies the product of conception dies early and is expelled from the uterus. In this event, termed spontaneous abortion, an individual existence ends almost immediately after onset. In observing such examples of life ended after only a brief flicker, we wish to know first whether the abortion can be traced to an abnormal condition of the ovum. We ask next whether the responsible deviation resides in the ovum from the beginning of the pregnancy or whether it is induced in the embryo by unfavorable conditions in the mother's body.

Before 1949 no concrete answers to these questions were available. In that year Drs. Arthur Hertig and John Rock published the results of their remarkable studies at the Boston Free Hospital for Women and the Carnegie Institute of Washington.[4] They examined microscopically twenty-eight implanted ova from the first sixteen days of pregnancy. These ova were found in the uteri of women who had to undergo hysterectomies for various medical reasons. None of the patients had missed a menstrual period, and in no instance had the diagnosis of pregnancy been made before surgery.

Hertig and Rock interpreted twelve of the twenty-eight ova as abnormal. In four instances the abnormalities were sufficiently severe to suggest that the pregnancies were destined for probable early abortion, and three cases were regarded as certain abortions. The ratio of the candidates for certain early abortion to the total sample was close to the 10 percent rate that is generally accepted for spontaneous abortions. The evidence from this investigation justified the belief that the conditions responsible for an early end to new life are inherent in the fertilized ovum.

Using tissue from spontaneous abortions, geneticists later tried to determine whether the fatal defect of the ovum was associated with chromosome abnormalities. At about the same time that Hertig and Rock published their pioneer work, other investigators developed the fundamental methods of chromosomal analysis. In this technique the cells first must be grown in tissue culture; the chromosomes subsequently are separated by immersion in hypotonic salt solution, a fluid having less dissolved material than the cell. This procedure made it possible to stain the chromosomes and view their microscopic details.

With the new techniques came rapid progress in the understanding of hereditary conditions. White blood cells were easy to grow in culture, but tissue cells were also suitable. Researchers found that they could use samples from aborted embryos or from the placenta, the tissue that mediates the exchange of vital substances between the blood of the mother and that of the embryo. Dr. David H. Carr at the University of Western Ontario examined tissue cultures from thirty-five spontaneous abortions and six stillborn infants. Fourteen days after the beginning of the cultures, they indicated chromosome abnormalities in eight cases.

Subsequent studies of early abortions made use of technical refinements. When subjected to special staining procedures, certain areas of the chromosomes stain more intensely than adjacent regions. This method makes the chromosomes appear "banded" and gives each of the forty-six chromosomes a characteristic pattern. With the aid of the banding technique, Drs. Dianne McConnell and David Carr from Canada's McMaster University Medical Center at Hamilton identified defects or irregular arrangements of chromosomes in sixteen of twenty-seven aborted tissue specimens.[5] The incidence of chromosomal deviations in spontaneous abortions is now generally believed to be 30 percent, or possibly higher.

The improved methods of chromosomal analysis are applicable also to the evaluation of couples with a history of recurrent abortions. Examples of such investigations are the reports by Dr. Morton Stenchever of the Utah College of Medicine[6] and Dr. Michael Mennuti at the University of Pennsylvania.[7] Their studies indicate a balanced chromosome translocation, Stenchever's finding it in one parent in 30 percent of spontaneous abortions, whereas Mennuti's found it in 14 percent of the couples. When the parents' chromosomes are normal, those of the offspring may still be deranged by errors during the division of the sperm cell or the ovum.

The relation of specific genes to inherited physical conditions was well established by the mid-1950s. There was abundant information about their distribution on the chromosomes, but the chemical composition of the genes was unknown. It was even questionable whether they had physical properties, although it had been proposed much earlier that the genes are material particles actually lying in and forming a part of the chromosomes with which they grow.

The chemistry of the genes and the mechanism that accounts for their replication were projects receiving investigators' highest priority. The breakthrough came in 1953 when James Watson, Francis Crick, Maurice Wilkins, and their colleagues identified the structure of deoxyribonucleic acid (DNA).[8] This substance is the genetic material of all cells and carries the genetic code. It consists of two chains of nucleotide bases that are held together by hydrogen bonds. Nucleotides are phosphoric esters of purine-carbohydrate compounds that are derived from hydrolysis of nucleic acid. The nucleotides of the DNA molecule are adenine, thymine, guanine, and cytosin. The chains are twisted about each other in the shape of a double helix. Replication occurs through new strands of DNA that form when the cell divides.

The four nucleotides of the helix are arranged in different sequences. Their combinations, called codons, represent genetic instructions that are passed from one generation to the next. Each codon is a combination of three adjacent nucleotide bases. The genetic code, comprising sixty-four triplet codons, contains all instructions to control the development and functions of the organism. The codons play this crucial role because each of them specifies the formation of one of the twenty amino acids that together constitute the protein substance of the body.

Although the genetic code resides in the nucleus of the cell, its specifications are transmitted to the cytoplasm by a messenger, ribonucleic acid (RNA). Within the cytoplasm the instructions of the genetic code regulate the synthesis of the amino acids and thus control the composition of the protein molecules. These in turn determine the physical characteristics and the functions of both the individual cells and the entire organism.

The discovery of the DNA structure brought the Nobel Prize to Watson, Crick, and Wilkins in 1962. The key to vital genetic problems had been found, and beyond this promise lay the conviction that the essence of life itself could be expressed in the precise terms of chemical analysis. It was Watson's belief that the discovery of DNA would soon enable us to understand all the basic features of the living state.[9]

That abnormal body chemistry can be inherited had become clear at the onset of the twentieth century through the work of Sir Archibald Garrod.[10] In 1903 he was the first to describe an inborn error of metabolism in which the lack of a specific gene is responsible for the absence of the enzyme that the gene controls. The enzyme deficiency in turn causes the failure of a specific biological reaction. In alkaptonuria an abnormal substance, homogentisic acid, causes discoloration of body tissues. The condition is due to a defect in the oxidation of homogentisic acid, the metabolic product of the amino acids phenylalanine and tyrosine. Garrod correctly attributed this metabolic deviation to the congenital lack of a specific enzyme, homogentisic acid oxidase. Other metabolic disorders, including phenylketonuria (see chap. 7), were later recognized as hereditary enzyme defects as well.

There is indeed a chemical individuality, as Garrod indicated. Just as anatomical traits are inherited, so are the chemical characteristics of the organism controlled by the genetic code. This control is not limited to enzymatic reactions or other phases of the metabolism. Dr. Linus Pauling proved in 1949 that sickle-cell anemia is due to a single change in the amino acid sequence of the hemoglobin molecule caused by a recessive mutant gene.[11] If the abnormal gene is matched with a normal gene on the corresponding chromosome, the condition is heterozygous and the affected person shows only the sickling *trait*, which has no appreciable ill effect. Homozygous persons have two abnormal genes and are victims of sickle cell *disease*, with recurrent bouts of severe anemia.

The contributions of the chemists and physicists have opened new vistas in medical genetics. The Mendelian laws, the structure of the chromosomes, and the distribution of the genes are as valid as ever, but this knowledge has been enriched by the new discipline of molecular genetics. We can now define a gene as a segment of DNA that produces a corresponding segment of messenger RNA; in turn this RNA is translated into a specific portion of body protein. Dr. François Jacob, who received the Nobel Prize for his work on messenger RNA, expressed the meaning of the new genetics as follows: "Heredity is described today in terms of information, messages and code. The reproduction of an organism has become that of its constituent molecules. This is not because each chemical species has the ability to produce copies of itself, but because the structure of the macro-molecules is determined down to the last detail by sequences of four chemical radicals contained in the genetic heritage."[12]

The new knowledge has made it easier for us to understand the concept of mutations. These sudden jumps of genetic properties represent changes in the DNA molecule ranging from tiny to large. The smallest are subtle alterations at one point of the chromosome (point mutations). They cause no visible change in the appearance of the chromosome and involve a derangement in the nucleotide sequence of the DNA complex that may result in the substitution of a single amino acid within a protein molecule. Large mutations result from the breakage of chromosomes, removal of a small part of a chromosome (deletion), its duplication, or its inversion. Fragmentation of an X chromosome, for instance, causes the "fragile X syndrome," which is associated with mental retardation.

The detailed knowledge of the causes of mutations is vital to our understanding of disease, for they account not only for congenital disorders but also for the inherited disposition to diseases that develop in adult life. Radiation and other environmental agents can interfere with the synthesis of DNA in a sex cell. The result may be simply an altered sequence of two nucleotides, but this derangement is sufficient to change the nature of a gene that controls important physical or functional traits of future organisms. Our ability to cope with the environment depends on the structure of DNA, which is itself influenced by the environment.

As soon as we realize this dual dependence, we ask which specific outside agents can cause mutations. A comprehensive knowledge of these mutagens is invaluable, since it would help us to minimize harmful alterations of our genetic material. This knowledge is just beginning to be available, although its usefulness is limited. The evidence suggests that many environmental agents can damage the chromosomes. If this damage occurs in the tissue cells (autosomes), it may lead to abnormal growth of tissues that eventually can result in cancer. These autosomal mutations are not hereditary but are limited to the affected individuals. If the chromosomal deviations are induced in sex cells, they lead to mutant genes that are passed on to future generations.

A multitude of chemical substances, natural as well as synthetic, are known to induce mutations in laboratory animals and bacteria. It would be ideal to know which of these substances can affect human chromosomes and thereby have a list of mutagenic agents to avoid. Since valid tests of this type are not yet available, we can be guided only by evidence that, although not conclusive, is strongly suggestive. Such evidence may be obtained by analyzing population surveys that demonstrate increases in stillbirths or congenital defects and suggest a rise in the mutation rate. Epidemiologists can subsequently attempt to correlate this heightened mutagenic activity with the introduction of a specific external agent.

Results of human population surveys, coupled with experimental observations on microbes and animals, give us lists of likely mutagens, most of which are also suspected of being carcinogens. Several comprehensive tabulations of this nature are available. One of them is the work of Dr. Lawrence Fishbein from the National Center of Toxicological Research.[13] Similar research was conducted by J. Kline, Z. Stein, and M. Susser.[14]

Among the natural mutagens, the aromatic hydrocarbons are the best known. Benzo(a)pyrene, which has been found to be mutagenic in the *Drosophila* fly, is the most important representative of this group. The sources of this substance are numerous and manifold. They include soil, air, water, gasoline engines, rubber tire dust, cigarette smoke, mineral oil, wax, and certain foods and beverages. Pollution is the main source of benzopyrene in soil and water, and we realize what the term *natural* means: the culprit occurs in nature, but its dangerous concentrations are due mainly to our own activities. Other members of the natural group are the nitrosamines, sulfur oxides, and nitrogen oxides.

The synthetic potential mutagens include chlorinated hydrocarbons (trichlorethylene, vinylchloride, and carbontetrachloride), formaldehyde, and ethylene oxide. Metal products, particularly those that contain lead, mercury, or arsenic, are also in this group. DDT and some other pesticides are believed to be mutagenic, as are certain drugs, among which the alkylating agents (bisulfan, chlorambucil, and cyclophosphamide) are associated with chromosomal damage. They are at present employed in cancer chemotherapy and illustrate the need for taking calculated risks in using synthetic agents until safer ones are available. Controlled application and proper precautions will minimize the damage that these substances cause.

The recent advances in genetics have contributed substantially to our concept of disease. In the light of the new knowledge, Bernard's *milieu intérieur* is now seen as a product of the genetic code. Its physical makeup and chemical composition are determined by the DNA of the ovum and sperm cell at the time of conception. Minimal deviations from the normal code may seriously impair the organism's vital metabolic functions.

The environment can alter the genetic code by causing mutations and possibly also by interfering with the normal separation of the chromosomes during the meiosis of the sperm cell or the ovum. The conflict between the inner system and the environment has a lasting effect that extends through generations and may mark any newly conceived organism with the stamp of disease. We need no longer wonder whether life begins with the perfect state of complete harmony between the internal system and the environment. Experience tells us that this state exists only as an ideal. Instead of being biologically perfect, the new organism contains inherited imperfections that place its inner system in immediate jeopardy.

In addition to facing possible inherited disadvantages, the new life is exposed to disease-causing hazards coming from the outside while still in the womb. Although the impact of the environment on any unborn creature began long ago with the modification of the genes by external mutagens, it continues after conception. Compared with the preconceptional phase, the intrauterine stage is extremely short, but it is subject to a host of potential influences. These constitute the prenatal environment, which is mediated by the maternal tissues and the placenta.

External factors that affect the fetus are not only numerous but are also markedly varied. Drugs, infections, and radiation are their main categories. The conflict with the environment may first lead to disease of the mother and affect the fetus secondarily. Maternal diabetes mellitus causes metabolic conditions that adversely affect the fetus. The high glucose level of the mother's blood is only one of the deviations that interfere with the intrauterine development in such a situation. Stillbirths are relatively frequent in pregnancies complicated by diabetes, and the infants of diabetic mothers are often overweight and may have congenital anomalies of organs or tissues. These babies are at risk also for respiratory distress syndrome, which is a common cause of neonatal death.

Aside from diabetes, certain other conditions make the intrauterine environment unfavorable for the developing fetus. If the mother has sickle-cell disease, an inadequate supply of oxygen will threaten the infant's life. Depending on the magnitude of the oxygen deficit, the baby may be stillborn or subject to growth retardation.

The causative agent of such disorders often has little effect on the mother but is devastating to the infant. This discrepancy is well illustrated by certain infections that complicate pregnancy. The timing of the infection in relation to the stage of the pregnancy frequently determines whether the fetus is vulnerable. Syphilis has long been recognized as a disease that can be transmitted from the mother to the unborn child. The causative spirochete, *Treponema pallidum,* is the outside agent that infects the mother. The disease has three distinct stages, but the fetus is vulnerable mainly during the first two.

We realize here some of the intricacies in the causation of disease. The developing individual makes contact with the hazards of the outside world through the placenta and the tissues of the mother. Early diagnosis of infection affords an opportunity for protecting the infant by adequate treatment of the mother. We have a chance to neutralize the harmful forces in the environment before they can touch the new life and cause stillbirth, neonatal death, or congenital disease.

The term *TORCH syndrome* applies to certain infections that are life-threatening in the newborn, whereas the mother usually suffers no serious harm. *TORCH* stands for toxoplasmosis, rubella, cytomegalic disease, and herpes. The manifestations of these diseases may be so mild that the mother need not be aware of any past or recent infection. The diagnosis therefore often depends on the judicious use of laboratory tests.

Humans acquire toxoplasmosis by eating rare meat or by having contact with sick cats. The causative organism is a parasite, *Toxoplasma gondii,* and the infection is virtually asymptomatic in adults.* In the fetus toxoplasmosis may be fatal or cause severe damage to the eyes and the nervous system. The risk to the infant depends on the timing of the infection. Transmission is most common when the mother acquires the disease during the last third of her pregnancy, but infections occurring during the first third are more likely to result in severe damage to the infant's brain.

Rubella (German measles) is usually a mild illness, and an expectant mother may not even know that she has been infected. Transplacental

---

*Except in immunodeficiency diseases, especially AIDS.

passage of the virus during the early stage of pregnancy, however, often leads to a complex of congenital defects consisting mainly of low birth weight, heart disease, and impaired hearing.

The cytomegalovirus is seldom responsible for serious problems in adults. Furthermore, it is often present in the fetus without ill effects, but in some instances it may lead to mental retardation and deafness.

The herpes simplex virus causes ulcers or blisters on the skin and mucous membranes in adults. The genital tract is a common site of these lesions, and the infant may be infected while passing through the birth canal. Although in adults the herpes lesions are painful, tend to recur, and are resistant to treatment, they are not life-threatening. In infants the virus can cause an illness that begins a few days after birth and often ends with the baby's death in the second to fourth week of life. In addition, maternal herpes may be a risk factor before delivery. Dr. Thomas Lawley and his associates at the National Institutes of Health reviewed forty-one cases of women who had herpes during pregnancy.[15] There were eight premature deliveries, four stillbirths, and one spontaneous abortion. Herpes in pregnancy therefore constitutes a risk to the fetus, as well as a hazard to the newborn.

The infections of the TORCH category are examples that illustrate the action of environmental agents in pregnancy. It is typical that they involve the mother and the infant in different ways and that their effect is subject to timing. Since fetal tissues develop rapidly, a slight difference in the gestational age may be crucial to the impact of drugs, radiation, or infection.

Much of the fetal environment is imposed by the mother, who sometimes has the option of keeping away injurious substances. There is still no complete agreement on the effects of smoking and alcohol consumption during pregnancy, but there is good evidence that both may be harmful. Reduction of birth weight and retardation of the baby's growth have been attributed to maternal smoking. Heavy drinking has been associated with low birth weight, and some experts recognize a "fetal alcohol syndrome," which includes small size, facial deformities, and mental deficiency.

In most instances the mother is not aware of subjecting the fetus to a hostile environment. For example, radiation can penetrate the mother's tissues and directly damage the nervous system of the fetus. Mental retardation frequently results and may be accompanied by visible malformations, the most common of which is an undersized brain (microceph-

aly). Injury to the fetus occurs mainly when the mother receives relatively heavy radiation in the course of treatment for cancer. This form of treatment is now usually postponed for the duration of the pregnancy.

More common than the direct impact of an outside agent on the fetus
is the transplacental passage of harmful substances. The placenta is composed of fetal and maternal tissues, and its function is the exchange of
nutrients and waste products. It is spongy tissue full of small blood vessels and is attached to the lining of the uterus. It communicates with the
infant through the blood vessels in the umbilical cord. The placenta is,
therefore, the interface where the infant's internal system makes contact
with the outside world.

Transplacental passage is possible not only for vital substances but also
for drugs and toxic chemicals, including carcinogens. Many substances
that may pose a threat to the unborn child are tolerated by the mother
without any ill effects. The hazard to the fetus may remain unrecognized
until birth or, in some cases, until many years later. In 1961 an unusual
number of severely deformed infants were born in Europe. The outstand-
ing feature was phocomelia, a condition that is characterized by many
severe defects, including deformed extremities that resemble the flippers
of a seal. The cause of the tragedy was finally traced to thalidomide, a new
tranquilizer that had been prescribed frequently for pregnant women.

Less dramatic, but perhaps more intriguing, was the role of diethylstil-
besterol (DES), a synthetic product with properties similar to estrogen.
Dr. Arthur Herbst and his associates at the Vincent Memorial Hospital
in Boston observed a rare cancer of the vagina in eight young women who
had been born in New England hospitals between 1946 and 1951.[16] A
retrospective investigation revealed that the mothers of all these young
patients had received DES during the first trimester of their pregnancies.
This medication was at that time accepted as preventive treatment when
bleeding during pregnancy signaled an impending abortion.

The observations of the Boston group suggested that DES traversed the
placenta and acted on the developing reproductive tract of the fetus. The
result in most cases was a minor abnormality of the genital organs, but
in rare instances vaginal cancer appeared in the offspring during the second or third decade of life.

When interviewed in 1980 Dr. Herbst had collected additional information. He estimated that the risk of acquiring the cancer was slightly less
than 0.1 percent for women who had been exposed to DES during their
fetal development. The story of the "DES babies" increases our under-

standing of the effect the environment can have on the organism. DES is a product of human invention. It was given to pregnant women for medical reasons. There was no evidence of any damage to the mothers, nor did the infants show any signs of disease. Nonetheless, there were subtle changes in the tissues that formed the genital tract, and in a few of the offspring these changes were conducive to cancer.

What we have learned about the complications of DES makes us question whether we will discover more agents that are innocuous to the adult but act imperceptibly on the tissues of the fetus. We must be alert to this possibility, for the example of DES has taught us that an abnormal condition might begin before birth and remain latent for years.

Even if characteristic abnormalities occur in a number of newborn infants within a circumscribed geographic area, the causative agent need not be obvious. Minimata disease is named after the Minimata Bay area of Japan. In the 1950s and 1960s cerebral palsy developed there in forty babies whose mothers remained well. The outbreak was eventually traced to a mercury compound that had been dumped into the bay and was ingested by the fish. The mercury in the fish, when eaten by a pregnant woman, reached the nervous system of the fetus through transplacental passage. Dried stumps of the umbilical cords of some of the victims had been preserved. Analysis of the cords by two Tokyo scientists, Drs. Susumu Nishigaki and Masazumi Harada, proved that the tissues had a high content of mercury.[17]

In the study of congenital defects, the importance of a causative complex rather than a single cause is readily apparent. Dr. Rolf Terge Lie of the University of Bergen, Norway, analyzed the records of 371,933 women from 1967 through 1989.[18] He found that 2.5 percent of these women had given birth to babies each of whom had one defect. These mothers of affected first infants were 2.4 times as likely as other women to have a second child with the same defect. The risk became considerably less if the women moved to a different location between the first and second pregnancy. A different combination of harmful occupational and environmental agents was likely to be responsible for the difference in the rates of risk.

From the moment of its conception the human organism is subject to physical deviations. The individual may be marked for disease by the genetic code or may come to harm while still in the uterus. In either case the new life is either visibly affected or carries the seed of disease without showing it. Contact with the environment is inseparable from biological existence. The fetus is shielded from the outside world but cannot escape the effect of hazardous substances that have entered the mother's blood. In rare instances the mother may be the source of harmful antibodies that endanger her own offspring. In erythroblastosis of the newborn, the mother's immune system responds to the Rh factor of the baby and causes severe damage to the infant's red blood cells (see chap. 7). The antagonism between the external milieu and the individual could hardly be shown more strikingly than by this example. In its early stage life is subject to the adverse action of the maternal tissues on which it depends for shelter and nourishment.

The concept of disease as the result of a conflict with the environment holds true for any period in the life of the individual, but the different periods vary from each other in the unit's susceptibility to different agents. External conditions that are right for a healthy young adult may be fatal to an octogenarian. A prematurely born infant is vulnerable to environmental factors that are normal for mature babies because the functioning systems of the premature infant cannot cope adequately.

Prematurity is particularly hazardous to the respiratory system. The blood's absorption of oxygen takes place in the air sacs of the lungs, where the inhaled air is in contact with a network of minute blood vessels. This intricate process requires a surfactant, a complex lipoprotein that is rich in highly saturated lecithins. The premature lung, being deficient in surfactant, cannot function properly. The clinical result of this defect is the respiratory distress syndrome that is responsible for approximately 20 percent of all neonatal deaths. Drs. Philip Farrell and Richard Zachman from the Wisconsin Perinatal Center in Madison report an incidence of the syndrome in 75 percent of infants born at less than thirty weeks gestation.[19] The syndrome appears in 22 percent of infants born at thirty-three to thirty-four weeks and 0.5 percent of infants carried to term.

When we consider the enormous number of changes that must occur before the new individual can take a breath, we understand that a few weeks or even days in the length of gestation can be crucial. The formation of organs and the shaping of the entire body take place during the first three months. Maturation of tissues and developing of body functions subsequently follow a crowded schedule until the pregnancy has gone to term.

Conception, birth, and death are three events so profound that our minds cannot penetrate their secrets. The biological existence of the individual begins as soon as the union of two sex cells provokes the growth and differentiation of the body cells. From its inception the new life has to interact with its surroundings. For a period of nine months it can meet this challenge only with the aid of its maternal connection. The mother has to eat for it, breathe for it, and generally provide a protective envelope against the raw environment.

Birth means the sudden loss of maternal mediation and the onset of independent functions. Coping with the environment becomes the prime task of the new organism. Food is no longer infused through the placental filter into the baby's bloodstream but must be swallowed and then assimilated in the digestive tract before it can be carried to the tissues. The lungs must inflate themselves with air to absorb the vital oxygen that hitherto had been supplied by the mother's circulation. Maternal immune antibodies against viruses and bacteria may remain in the infant's circulation for weeks or months, but eventually they disappear and the newborn must replace them.

These are but a few examples of the many functions that go into action without the benefit of a preparatory period. Whether the new life can continue depends on the success of this sudden changeover. At the same time, although the infant has become a separate unit, this unit still relies on support and shelter from the outside for a period of years. The child can digest suitable food, but he or she cannot obtain it without help and would perish unless protected against heat, cold, and other environmental elements.

Above all, the uniquely human way of surmounting adversities lags behind the physiological development. Decisions that are based on experience or calculations are the hallmark of human performance. When the individual has arrived at this level, he or she participates in the manipulation of the environment. This phase may mean purification or pollution, advancement or regression.

Even the fully developed organism is not self-sufficient, for it must obtain the necessities of life from the outside with the cooperation of others. Adaptation to the environment is decisive for survival. When the organism loses the ability to adapt, it can no longer interact properly with the external milieu, and its life comes to an end. In death there is a complete cessation of all biological functions. Maintenance of all body substance ends, and adaptation falls to the zero-level. Like the nature of life itself, the significance of birth and death remains a mystery to us. We can grasp only the importance of certain changing conditions, and among these adaptability is the easiest to understand.

The length of a person's life depends on his or her genetic material and on the prevailing external conditions. A combination of genes, personal decisions, and uncontrollable circumstances makes the difference between life and death for a number of decades.[20] After a certain maximal period, perhaps one hundred and twenty years in humans, the life of the unit comes to an end, regardless of any individual performance or external factors.

Most of us expect science to identify the cause or causes of aging and to find ways of retarding it. Research has given us some interesting theories about the mechanism of aging. These include animal experiments on the effect of caloric restriction and reduced body temperature, both of which prolong the animal's life span. Dr. Roy L. Walford and his co-workers at the UCLA School of Medicine proved that caloric restriction keeps the immune system intact longer and thereby postpones the onset of autoimmunity, which occurs more frequently as the body grows older.[21] When the immune system ages, it is apt to lose its ability to discriminate between self and nonself and might then attack the tissues it is supposed to protect.

We see a similarity between the beneficial effect of caloric restriction on immunity and its retarding action on arteriosclerosis. It is hard to escape the notion that the human body is attuned to a nutritional standard that is lower than what we ordinarily regard as desirable. Habit and comfort have obscured our natural judgment and make us consume more environmental products than we need.

Preferences and life-style are likely to be related to longevity in many different ways. Food selection varies from one person to another, as do physical activity, response to stress, exposure to carcinogens, and the like. Each of these differences is subject to individual decisions.

The potential length of a person's life is determined by biological conditions that are largely unknown at present. It lies within certain limits that are fairly specific for each species. There is good reason to believe that the limit of the life span is built into the genetic code. Genes that are advantageous to the survival of a species might carry with them lethal genes that make the continuation of life impossible after a certain age.

Some genetically determined diseases terminate life early and also cause signs of premature aging, particularly degeneration of blood vessels, cataracts, and presenile dementia. Down's syndrome and Werner's syndrome are examples of premature aging* associated with specific chromosomal aberrations.

One may assume the working theory that the genetic background of the average person is conducive to longevity if the organism can adjust itself to the environmental needs. Genotypes containing mutant genes necessitate specific adjustments beyond the average requirements. Phenylketonuria is an example of a condition that can be prevented by special diet (see chap. 7). This regime protects the body against the products of amino acids that it cannot metabolize properly. The fraction of the environment that serves as food must be modified in a particular way for persons with phenylketonuria.

We may expect to learn much more about genetic weaknesses of individuals and about methods that confer protection against specific defects. Such measures are likely to include diets, medication, and above all, avoidance of harmful environmental agents. Regardless of their precise nature, their essence will be the manipulation of the environment. Backed by firm evidence, we are entitled to predict a gradual reduction of diseases that terminate life relatively early. Each new decade will probably teach us more about living in harmony with the environment. In each decade to come, therefore, humankind should eliminate some causes of mortality.

This continued triumph over disease is not a victory over death but only a postponement of it. When we come to the question of the potential length of human life, we cannot make any reasonable predictions. The limit of longevity has shown no reliable signs of changing in the past, and we should not expect it to change in decades or even centuries to come. Regardless of how successful medical science might be in reducing mortality rates during the first one hundred years of life, it has nothing to offer when we approach the absolute and ultimate limit. We have many theoretical explanations of this limitation. The theory of "lethal genes" makes sense, for these would safeguard the species by preventing an overaged population that could no longer perform optimally.

Reports in the scientific publications have been of a preliminary nature when predicting the possible extension of life well beyond the hundred-year mark. The news media, nevertheless, have already relayed exciting speculations, and some men and women are already making plans for the extra years of their lives.

*Progeria is also a disease with severe signs of early aging and with death usually occurring in adolescence.

If their dreams should come true, however, these people will probably not be in good physical condition. The added years will subject their over-aged bodies to more wear and tear and will compound their physical discomfort. It will require many years of progress on all fronts of medicine before people could possibly enjoy any longevity of the magnitude that some might expect.

We must ask ourselves whether society would be able to meet the socioeconomic demands that a vastly larger number of much older citizens is bound to present. The gradual increase in the average life expectancy that occurred during the twentieth century is minimal compared with the added years believed possible by some scientists, but even now there are overwhelming problems related to the small extension of the life span. We can hardly expect the economy of any nation to improve magically to the extent that it will support the huge needs of many overaged people.

Will we ever learn the secret of our predestined cutoff from life? Will we be able to extend our allotted time by revitalizing the repair enzymes that are needed to keep our DNA, the stuff of life, from deteriorating? And if science should succeed in pushing the endpoint of our scale to one hundred and fifty years or beyond, would those very old people be able to cope with the exacting demands of an increasingly complex society?

We ask these questions while we stand before the Sphinx. And the Sphinx, its gaze fixed on infinity, remains silent.

6

Anatomy of Disease

I profess both to learn and to teach anatomy,
not from books but from dissections; not
from positions of philosophers but from the
fabric of nature.

—William Harvey, 1578–1657

The word *anatomy* comes from the
Greek and literally means "cutting up." We dissect the dead body to familiarize ourselves with its individual components. A similar plan is used to identify the parts of a mechanical device by dismantling it. Either procedure is expected to help us understand the relation of the various parts to one another and indicate possible causes of malfunction.

Anatomy has become synonymous with the composition or structure of an object. In addition to applying this term to physical entities, we may use it, loosely, for certain events or conditions, as in "anatomy of a murder."

When we want to explore the nature of disease, any effort to discern its essential parts seems doomed to failure. How can one determine the anatomy of a phantom that will often change from one vague shape to another? The phantom may not be visible or palpable, but it can be identified by the devastation it leaves behind in the bodies of its victims. A thorough knowledge of this damage is vital to any rational plan of cure or prevention.

Before the eighteenth century observations of this type were essentially limited to exterior inspection and yielded few specific clues. The plague, for instance, was known often to start with painful nodules in the groin that tended to swell and discharge pus. Similar changes occurred in non-fatal conditions that were not related to the plague.

Progress came at last when autopsies were performed and the findings evaluated in the light of the clinical information. The credit for initiating this method of investigation goes to Giovanni Battista Morgagni, professor of anatomy at the University of Padua in Italy from 1715 to 1771. During his long career he kept a careful record of his postmortem observations that were to become a milestone of medical research. Whereas others before him had performed autopsies to study normal anatomy, Morgagni correlated all visible deviations from the norm with any clinical information that was available in each case. He expressed the hope that his labors might shed light on the "sites and causes of diseases."[1]

Following this breakthrough the concept of an illness could be based on knowledge of its morbid anatomy. Pneumonia became known as severe congestion and consolidation of the lungs. Only after this understanding had been gained could new methods be devised that made possible an accurate diagnosis of pneumonia in the living. A similar approach led to a meaningful classification of many diseases and thereby opened ways to their diagnosis and treatment.

The study of the physical changes caused by disease is generally known as pathology. Whereas its pioneers relied on observations made with the naked eye, the use of the microscope soon brought immense advances by revealing tissue changes often indicative of specific diseases. Pathologists eventually could provide a diagnosis in the living by examining samples of excised tissue known as biopsies. Later yet, individual cells cast off from accessible sites were found to yield accurate information that proved valuable, particularly in the detection of cancer. The cell is not the smallest unit suitable for examination, since deviations of chromosomes and genes can be identified in many hereditary conditions.

In the two centuries since Morgagni first tried to find the sites and causes of diseases, medical science has made great progress toward that goal. In most instances diagnosis is no longer based entirely on the clinical evidence. It is usually established, or at least confirmed, by objective methods that make use of modern technology. After the sudden emergence of the acquired immunodeficiency syndrome (AIDS), for example, a reliable diagnostic test was soon available and the causative virus was identified.

Examination of biopsies will usually determine whether there is evidence of disease in a tissue sample and, if present, whether it is of the benign or malignant type. Malignancy means the presence of cancer. In that case the microscope will reveal a multitude of features in the shape, staining, and grouping of the cells that enable the observer to classify the specific type of cancer. This will provide the key to the optimal treatment. In any evaluation of malignancy it is important to judge its stage of advance. Cancer cells may still be confined to their site of origin. They may have invaded neighboring tissue, or they could even have been carried to distant sites by lymph fluid or blood.

Diseases other than cancer also have hallmarks that make their recognition by microscopic analysis possible. Characteristic tissue patterns are observed in many types of infection, and their classification can be finalized by identifying the causative agents. Minute particles of foreign matter, such as asbestos, can provide specific clues leading to the solution of difficult clinical problems.

Although microscopic examination identifies physical changes caused by disease, it has no monopoly in this field. X-ray examination and the newer, more sophisticated imaging methods are the primary tools with which the location, shape, and size of lesions are determined.

The detection of unsuspected disease is one of the prime objectives of modern medicine, since it will usually lead to treatment while the damage is still confined. To this purpose, screening methods have been devised that are painless, relatively simple, and cost effective. They are suited to repeated use in large groups of seemingly healthy persons. An example of mass screening is the microscopic examination of cells cast off from the uterine cervix* (the so-called Pap test). Only by this procedure, which is based on the pioneer work of Dr. George Papanicolaou, can routine screening identify the subclinical stages of cervical cancer.[2]

X-ray methods also pinpoint changes that are suspect of early cancer in many different locations. Perhaps the most impressive success of X-ray screening is the detection of early breast cancer by mammography. Many surveys have been conducted in different countries to assess the effective-

---

*The cervix is the portion of the womb, or uterus, that projects into the vagina.

ness of mammography in women who have no symptoms suggestive of breast cancer. A comprehensive review of these studies was made by the Council on Scientific Affairs of the American Medical Association. Its results afforded strong evidence that periodic mammographic screening of women over fifty years of age will reduce the rate of death from breast cancer. The more recent of these studies suggested a reduced mortality for younger women also.[3] The council concluded that mammography is currently the most effective method for detecting early breast cancers. If the mammography indicates malignancy, it must be followed by a biopsy before treatment is started.

The beginning of scientific medicine is usually attributed to the teachings of Hippocrates, who lived around 400 B.C. and who substituted rational judgment for ill-founded conjecture. But his time lacked the technology that is essential to any effective attack on disease. The contributions of science, particularly biology, chemistry, and physics, made possible those procedures that are indispensable to the physician. Accurate measurements of temperature, blood pressure, blood-cell count, and blood chemistry are but a few examples of basic diagnostic tools.

The instruments that are brought to the bedside and the multitude of laboratory tests, if combined with clinical evidence, represent much of the progress that has been made in recognizing many forms of disease. A more profound knowledge of any illness, however, is still unthinkable without the discipline of morbid anatomy. This type of investigation tells us about the nature of the disease process and its distribution within the body. What is apparent from the clinical impression may be only the tip of the iceberg. Pathology has taught us that an illness may have made inroads long before any symptoms appeared. This awareness established the concept of latent or subclinical disease, which is the basis for the life-saving methods of early detection.

The need to perform autopsies has not ceased. They are necessary not only for research but also for the critical review of whatever was done, or should have been done, while the patient was under medical care. The postmortem findings provide a measure of quality control, which is an essential requirement whenever human lives are at stake.[4]

Pathology, the anatomy of disease, had its beginning in the eighteenth century, but it did not exist in its present-day form for another hundred years, when Rudolf Virchow founded modern pathology. Before any investigation of morbid anatomy began, there had already been remarkable progress in studying the normal structure and function of the human body. Around the middle of the sixteenth century Andreas Vesalius had initiated modern anatomy by meticulous dissections and observations that he published in his fundamental work entitled *The Structure of the Human Body*.[5] Later in the same century William Harvey conceived the correct explanation of the circulation of the blood and outlined it in his treatise *The Motion of the Heart*.[6]

In any field of human endeavor we like to assume an orderly chain of progress, with each new achievement logically following its predecessors. This is an overly simplified view, since such straightforward advance is often complicated by chance observations leading to new ideas. The history of medicine abounds with discoveries that were not simply extensions of previously gained knowledge. Serendipity has played an important role in promoting science. The lucky find of an alert observer may lead to a sensational breakthrough. We owe the discovery of penicillin and the other antibiotics to the accidental contamination of a bacterial culture with a mold. Sir Alexander Fleming noted that the growth of the bacteria had been inhibited in a wide zone around the mold colony. He subsequently made an extract from the contaminant that proved highly successful in treating bacterial infections.

Regardless of all the weapons we have acquired for the fight against disease, we must have a thorough knowledge of its portal of entry, its trail of invasion, and the destruction at its sites of attack. Identification of the causative agent may then become possible and lead to a cure or preventive method. The legacies of Morgagni, Vesalius, and Harvey do not contain any prescriptions or curative surgical procedures, but they are vital to our understanding of disease. By actually seeing its telltale evidence, we may determine its mode of action. A painful swelling caused by infection is a sign of defense, but if this fails, it may be followed by fatal sepsis. Cells can change their behavior because of damage originating from the environment, such as bacteria, viruses, chemicals, or radiation. They may also react unfavorably to a lack of a substance they require for their maintenance that the environment usually supplies.

The exact type of the deviate reaction varies according to its cause and the properties of the host cells. These may swell, shrink, or become distorted. They may also display an excessive rate of division, which characterizes cancer cells and leads to the invasion of healthy tissue.

The anatomy of disease is basic to almost any specialty of medicine. This ongoing research has been rewarded by innumerable achievements in the diagnosis, treatment, and prevention of disease. Smallpox is now classified as eradicated. The plague and cholera have been reduced in incidence and made amenable to treatment. Nonetheless, the odds are against humankind's hope that disease may someday vanish from the earth entirely. One reason for skepticism is the possible emergence of new epidemics due to the activation or mutation of a dormant virus. Ironically, an even more ominous threat stems from our own attempts to improve the quality of our lives through a host of inventions. The innovations are not confined to industry but relate also to agriculture, nutrition, and many other fields of human endeavor, including medicine itself. Any new methods involve a potential tampering with the environment and have effects that cannot be anticipated. Our awareness of any new hazardous substances is often delayed for years. Lead, asbestos, hydrocarbons, and DDT are only a few examples of carcinogens or other disease-causing agents that were regarded as useful and harmless until their true natures were finally discovered. The smoking habit, which serves no useful purpose, lasted for centuries before its fatal nature was unmasked.

In times past ignorance made some people think of disease as a phantom that inflicted pain and death on its victims. Science has accomplished much since those dark days by coming closer to the true nature of the scourge. The phantom has been wounded, but like the Hydra of the Greek fable, it has many heads that can renew themselves when severed. Hercules, so the story goes, contrived to slay the monster by using a clever trick. Since medical science, unlike mythology, is not born of fantasy, we have little cause to look for another Hercules who will free us from the phantom of disease.

Although the enemy is still at large, we have learned much about its strategy and are steadily adding to our knowledge. We know the morbid anatomy of many diseases and have discovered their mechanisms of action. We have often identified their causative complexes and found effective remedies. Lest we become overly confident, however, we might look at the long list of ailments whose morbid anatomy has been explored but whose causes remain obscure, with no cures for them in sight. This holds true especially for many conditions of the nervous system. Parkinson's disease ("shaking palsy"), Alzheimer's disease (progressive dementia), and amyotrophic lateral sclerosis (Lou Gehrig's disease) are but a few sobering examples.

The research on Alzheimer's disease in particular demonstrates the importance of the causative complex rather than a single cause. Several substances are likely to affect the onset and the progress of this ailment.

Amyloid and other abnormal proteins are among these culprits. Geneticists, furthermore, have identified a "susceptibility gene" that promotes the progress of specific lesions in the nervous system of patients with Alzheimer's. The all-important principal cause seems to have escaped detection, however, and the causal complex has remained incomplete.

We cannot expect any regular sequence or timetable for research in medicine.[7] Sometimes it is only the last step in the chain of discovery that cannot be taken. The AIDS epidemic is typical of this frustrating situation. In a relatively short period of time after the emergence of this new scourge, research revealed its morbid anatomy and identified the HIV virus as its cause.[8] A reliable laboratory test for its diagnosis also became available soon. Nonetheless, although the number of AIDS patients is growing rapidly, science can hold out no promise of a cure in the foreseeable future, in spite of the passionate demands of the sufferers and the large sums of money provided by the government.

The practice of pathology is not ordinarily engaged in the direct care of patients, but it is indispensable to practicing physicians by helping them with the diagnosis, prognosis, and selection of treatment. Diagnosis is often determined by taking a biopsy, which is necessary in the evaluation of any neoplastic growth. From an adequate tissue sample a competent pathologist can usually decide whether a tumor is benign or malignant, from which normal tissue it has originated, and how aggressive it will be.

The examination of a biopsy may require special methods, such as sophisticated staining of tissue sections or viewing with the electron microscope for higher magnification. The most exciting technical advances, however, are based on the discoveries that have come from the exploration of the genome. Abnormal chromosomes may be the sites of mutant genes (oncogenes) that are responsible for the formation of certain neoplasms. The analysis of the content of DNA in the abnormal cells can be used to predict their rate of growth and thereby provide clues to the patient's prognosis.[9]

In the future a tumor might be identified according to the specific deviation of the normal DNA sequence at the critical position of one chromosome. This knowledge, perhaps in combination with other laboratory tests and clinical data, should indicate the diagnosis and important properties of the tumor. It might also tell us whether there is a hereditary tendency for this neoplasm to occur in coming generations.[10]

For practical purposes, information based on the examination of chromosomes, DNA, and RNA is not yet available in its complete form, but we are justified in expecting that it will become available in the future. We may even hope that it will come in the *near* future.

Our knowledge of the anatomy of disease has been immensely enriched since Morgagni published his pioneer work on the sites and causes of diseases. Present-day morbid anatomy has evolved into the exploration of any deviation from the normal in the body's tissues and cells, including all the known components of their nuclei. Laboratory tests can give us information on diseases of the metabolism, the blood, and the endocrine system. They can also identify the microorganisms and viruses that are responsible for infections.[11]

The possession of this knowledge imposes a great responsibility on the medical profession, as well as on the public. Physicians must exercise discipline in the judicious selection of diagnostic procedures instead of simply ordering a battery of tests. The public should cooperate with the doctors by refraining from demanding any new method that the news media might announce before it has been adequately tested. Without these restraints, medical facilities and personnel would be faced with an overwhelming workload.

The discoveries made by scientists can turn into either a boon for or a threat to humankind. Atomic energy is the striking proof of this double potential, but it holds true for less-momentous discoveries also. They are artificially produced, and the people decide on the manner in which they are used. Without strict controls there may be disaster rather than benefit. How we utilize these gifts from science is up to us.

7

Prevention:
Absolute and Limited

Preventives of evil are far better than remedies;
cheaper and easier of application, and surer in
result.

—Tryon Edwards, *The New Dictionary
of Thoughts*

The ultimate aim of humankind's approach to any evil is prevention. Speeches are made, books are written, and lectures given on the ways of keeping the great scourges of the world from occurring. There should be no war, no famine, no natural disasters, no poverty—and no disease. After centuries of research and lecturing, however, all these scourges are still with us.

If we want to dream of the perfect state of health, we must think of absolute prevention, which implies that the disease is not allowed to begin, even in its early stage. This has been accomplished in a number of conditions, as exemplified by the eradication of smallpox. There are nevertheless many conditions for which we must rely on limited prevention, attempting to stem the further course of the morbid process before it has caused any appreciable damage. This approach requires an awareness of "preclinical disease," which refers to a stage at which no symptoms or signs of any disease have become noticeable. This is accomplished by screening methods, such as the detection of subclinical diabetes by determination of the blood-glucose level or the early diagnosis of glaucoma by measuring the pressure within the eye.

Ideally, screening of this type should be made available periodically to large groups of the population. It should not require excessive funding, and it should lead to the early treatment of any condition that it uncovers.

A brilliant example of limited prevention is the early detection of cancer of the cervix by the so-called Pap smear, which is based on a method introduced by Dr. George N. Papanicolaou.[1] Subtle changes in the cells that are cast off from the cervix indicate malignancy or earlier, atypical features that may precede it. The smear may have to be repeated and may also have to be followed by a biopsy. If this screening method is carried out carefully, any cancer that might be present is usually detected in its preinvasive stage. Invasive cancer of the cervix was a dreaded and common disease before the advent of the Papanicolaou method, but the test subsequently lowered its incidence severely.

Not all efforts at limited prevention meet with the same success, since some are beset by problems of evaluation. After the first announcement of a new screening procedure in a scientific journal, the media often release the information to the public early on. Many persons will request their doctors to give them the immediate benefit of the new test, which might later be found to be ineffective after causing the patients to incur expenses and possibly to undergo unnecessary treatment. Even after a method of limited prevention has been successful for years, it may lose some or all of its usefulness due to changing conditions within the population or its environment. The control of tuberculosis by early recognition demonstrates this unfortunate turn of events.

Tuberculosis, the "White Plague" of centuries past, proved essentially resistant to general health measures until an efficient treatment became available. The incidence was higher among the poor who lived in crowded and unhygienic conditions, but the affluent class was not immune, and no particular way of life could promise freedom from tuberculosis. Institutions such as the Berghof Sanitarium in Thomas Mann's novel *The Magic Mountain* were, according to the author, feasible only in a capitalist economy. "Only under such a system," Mann explains, "was it possible for patients to remain there year after year at the family's expense."[2]

Nevertheless, one after the other they vacated their expensive rooms and their assigned places at the dinner table: "The gaps in the dining room were partly due to the exercise of choice; but some of them yawned in a particularly hollow manner—as, for instance, at Dr. Blumenkohl's place— he being dead."[3]

Morbidity and mortality from tuberculosis began to decline steadily after Selman Waksman's introduction of the antibiotic streptomycin in 1943.[4] Before that time patients were told to avoid dampness and cold climate and to keep up their strength with ample rest and good food. In spite of these measures, the devastating effect of the tubercle bacillus remained virtually unchecked in the lung tissue and also in other locations, such as the bones, joints, and central nervous system. Thomas Mann noted, "White blood corpuscles were attracted to the seat of the evil; the breaking-down proceeded apace; and meanwhile the soluble toxin released by the bacteria had already poisoned the nerve centers, the entire organization was in a state of high fever, and staggered—so to speak with heaving bosom—toward dissolution."[5]

When streptomycin and, later, other drugs were found to be effective in the treatment of tuberculosis, the death rate from this disease dropped to 1.4 per 100,000. The Swiss sanatoriums became hotels.

The fact that the advance of the tuberculous process could be checked and often arrested constituted an important measure of limited prevention. Close contacts of the patients, furthermore, could benefit from early diagnosis and prophylactic treatment, and inactive "dormant" tuberculosis could be kept from spreading. Our sense of security, however, was shattered in the 1980s by a menacing rise in the incidence of tuberculosis that came in the wake of the AIDS epidemic.[6] AIDS (acquired immunodeficiency syndrome) is caused by a virus that destroys the immunity of its victims. The tubercle bacillus is among the microorganisms that invade the AIDS patient's tissues virtually unchecked. The cases of active tuberculosis increased rapidly in number, and the traditional type of medication no longer afforded protection. This alarming reversal was found to be due to the emergence of drug-resistant strains of the bacillus that had developed in the immunodeficient patients. Subsequently the resistant strains affected persons who were free of AIDS but had dormant, or subdued, tuberculosis.

The return of the White Plague was an off-shoot of a new epidemic for which no remedy was available. This turn of events illustrates the enigmatic nature of disease. We do not know why the human immunodeficiency virus (HIV) suddenly began to terrorize large groups of the world's population. We do know that the avoidance of certain practices, such as intravenous drug abuse, might have minimized its spread, but the human factor stymied compliance with public health measures.

The frustrating experience with the control of tuberculosis should not diminish our confidence in the validity of limited prevention. We must regard it as a method that usually, although not always, stops disease in its tracks before the patient has come to harm and often before he or she is aware of any problem. Screening of symptom-free people has stood the test of time and has firmly established its value in the detection of diabetes, high blood pressure, and cancer of the cervix. The periodic performance of mammograms has also been accepted as a routine health measure, although it lacks some of the simplicity of the older methods. New methods are subject to long-term follow-up before they can be recommended to the public without any reservations. An evaluation period of several years is often necessary before the test can be regarded as practical and cost effective. Without watchfulness and a critical attitude, we would eventually have a long list of procedures of questionable value that could be expensive and time-consuming for the patients.

Some methods of prevention will eventually have to be discarded, or perhaps limited to persons with known risk factors, such as belonging to a family with a high incidence of certain malignant tumors. In spite of these restrictions, limited prevention has reached a large number of men, women, and children and has saved many of them from the full impact of serious illnesses. This contribution by the medical profession ranks second only to the complete avoidance of disease.

Absolute prevention is the most desirable measure in health preservation, for it denies disease a chance to get a start. This form of preventive medicine is practiced more commonly than most of us realize. It is used to great advantage in dealing with the world of the parasites. Diseases caused by animal parasites, or transmitted by animal carriers, can be prevented by sanitation. They are rare in geographic locations enjoying good public health facilities.

Medical students must memorize all that is known about trichinosis, but few of them will ever diagnose or treat this condition. Humans acquire trichinosis principally by eating improperly cooked meat from infested hogs. Infestation of these animals comes from their ingestion of pork scraps or rats containing the larvae of the parasite. Prevention is accomplished by adequately inspecting meat, thoroughly cooking pork before it is eaten, and heating the garbage that is fed to the hogs.

Trichinosis is but one example of the many parasitic infestations that can be kept away from humans. All these infestations present potentially serious diseases that we need not contract. Avoidance has eliminated the need for treatment. Similar progress has been made against hookworm disease, tapeworm infestations, and amebiasis. All these ills have been markedly reduced in incidence through improved personal and environmental hygiene.

Control of insect-borne conditions is more difficult, but these have nevertheless been greatly reduced in their epidemic form. Malaria, typhus, yellow fever, and plague, although not eradicated, no longer hold the terror of years past. Absolute prevention is achieved mainly through the extermination of the insect vectors—mosquitoes, flies, rat-fleas, and lice.

Control of parasites has its problems, such as the use of insecticides that exert potential toxic effects on humans and animals. Furthermore, measures aimed at the improvement of rural conditions may unwittingly promote the spread of disease. Irrigation of farmlands in Egypt, for instance, led to an increase of snails that transmit schistosomiasis, a chronic affliction mainly involving the urinary bladder and sometimes terminating in cancer.

When preventive parasitology fails, the most common cause of this failure is the human reaction—or more accurately, inaction. The method may be available but not used properly. Europe, for instance, is virtually free of malaria. The Americas also have markedly decreased its incidence within their borders, but the disease continues to be prevalent in the equatorial areas of the world. Faust, Russell, and Jung state that "the World Health Organization reports Europe to be almost free of malaria, and the Pan-American Health Organization is actively campaigning to eradicate the disease from the Americas." They state further, "In the less developed countries, particularly in Africa, the eradication of malaria remains a formidable task."[7]

Absolute prevention protects us against parasites of which many of us have never heard and against the bacteria or viruses that they carry. It keeps us safe from food poisoning caused by the *Staphylococcus, Salmonella,* and the deadly *botulinus* organisms. Sanitary rules for handling, processing, and canning food have eliminated these infections except for isolated outbreaks.

Asepsis, a form of supercleanliness, is the principle of absolute prevention as applied to surgery. Postoperative infections cannot occur if the instruments, gloves, gowns, and dressings used are germ-free. Surgeons have adopted the best preventive method to avoid iatrogenic complications.

In obstetrics the conscientious avoidance of contamination proved to be the solution to the enigma of childbed fever, "the curse of Eve." Even before the responsible microbes had been identified, Dr. Oliver Wendell Holmes proposed in 1843 that the disease was "so far contagious as to be frequently carried from patient to patient by physicians and nurses."[8]

Four years later Dr. Ignaz Semmelweiss announced in Vienna that puerperal fever was induced blood poisoning and could be avoided by simple precautions that keep the contagion away from the patients. Like the surgeons, the obstetricians induced fatal iatrogenic complications until their procedures were made safe by preventive measures.

A characteristic feature of absolute prevention is its independence from the ways of nature. Progress in medicine is often based on functions that we borrow from nature and adjust to our own purpose. Penicillin, for instance, is normally produced by molds and serves to protect them against bacteria. Usually, humankind observes nature, analyzes what it sees, then takes what it believes to be useful. Absolute prevention, however, is our original brainchild. It has no natural precedent after which it is patterned. To kill parasites or microbes by boiling is strictly a human invention, and so is avoidance of contamination by aseptic methods.

Vaccination, one of our most powerful tools against disease, is not really an absolute method. The virus or the bacteria are not kept from us but are rendered harmless by immune antibodies that result from the vaccination. Unlike absolute prevention, vaccination borrows its principle from nature. It tricks nature by causing the disease to appear in a mild form. The body reacts by producing specific antibodies that eventually protect it against the infection.

The first successful trick of this kind was performed by Edward Jenner on May 14, 1796. According to his own account, he inoculated a healthy boy about eight years old with fluid taken from a sore on the hand of a dairy maid who was infected by her master's cow. "What renders the cow-pox virus so extremely singular," wrote Jenner two years later, "is that the person who has been thus affected is forever-after secure from the infection of the smallpox."[9]

Almost one hundred years later Pasteur made use of Jenner's discovery and introduced the method of vaccination against rabies.[10] This meant that prevention was possible for a disease that until then had been invariably fatal. Subsequently, active immunization was perfected against a host of diseases, notably diphtheria, tetanus, and poliomyelitis. (In passive immunization antibodies are transferred to an infected person by injecting the serum of a vaccinated animal. This method confers immediate protection that is short-lived, however.)

Vaccination is a choice example of medical progress. It may be called near-absolute prevention, but it lacks the simplicity and the quiet efficiency of the truly absolute method. Like any medical innovation that promises freedom from a dread disease, it is not always accepted with enthusiasm. The public, in fact, is often slow to accept a new vaccine. Furthermore, it will lose interest in a successful immunization program when the incidence of the disease has declined. A 1975 audit of private-practice physicians revealed that only 40 percent of two-year-olds were adequately immunized against polio.

This reluctance to make full use of an obvious boon to health is difficult to explain, since several factors influence people's decisions. One of these problems derives from the potential complications that, although rare, can befall any immunization program with disastrous results. Contamination of the vaccine may lead to severe illness or death. Even an uncontaminated vaccine may have poorly understood side effects that can trigger a series of dangerous changes in the central nervous system and may terminate in paralysis. These rare adverse reactions receive wide publicity, which results in large-scale avoidance of the facilities for vaccination.

The case of the swine influenza vaccine is an example of the ramifications that may stem from new vaccination projects. First came the controversy about the decision to initiate this program against a strain of influenza that had been identified in only a few isolated cases but nevertheless might have caused an epidemic later. The federal government decided to act, and the vaccine was manufactured at public expense.

The project was doomed when some of the immunized persons fell victim to Guillain-Barré (G-B) syndrome, a form of paralysis that often disappears after a number of weeks. It is sometimes permanent but rarely fatal. The overall rate of this syndrome was significantly higher among recipients of the swine flu vaccine than in nonrecipients (13.3 cases per 1 million for the former and 2.6 per 1 million for the latter). This difference in the rates between the vaccinated and unvaccinated population was regarded as statistically significant. Claims approaching 1 billion dollars were lodged against the government on behalf of the persons who suffered from G-B syndrome. The final condemnation of the project came when no epidemic of swine influenza materialized, although the vast majority of the population had not taken the vaccine. The stage was set for severe criticism with more political than medical overtones.

Low immunization rates cannot be blamed solely on adverse publicity; sometimes they result from caution or skepticism of physicians. Any new program that has been proved reasonably safe and effective must be implemented by the medical profession, but doctors have to be convinced of the method's safety, value, and necessity before they will recommend it to their patients. Hospitals, clinics, and health centers must decide in staff meetings whether to employ the program at all. If they decide to do so, the specific rules of application still remain to be determined, for a vaccine often is given only to selected groups of persons who are at high risk for the illness against which protection is conferred. The elderly and those afflicted with chronic ailments are examples of high-risk categories.

Events accompanying or following the release of a new vaccine illustrate the problems that the developers of the program must face. A polyvalent pneumococcal vaccine effective against fourteen types of pneumonia-causing bacteria became commercially available in February 1978. Of three health centers surveyed three months later, one had immunized 90 percent of high-risk patients; the second had stocked the vaccine but had not yet administered it; and the third had neither ordered the vaccine nor contemplated doing so. This erratic response to a new preventive method shows that the medical profession's attitude toward immunization procedures is not immediately enthusiastic. The vaccine eventually gained recognition by the medical profession, but its use is still limited by its cost. (The valency of the vaccine had been increased from fourteen to twenty-three types of the bacteria by 1994.)

Two centuries after Jenner's discovery, the specter of smallpox epidemics has disappeared.[11] In December 1979 the World Health Organization concluded that smallpox eradication had been achieved throughout the world. There followed a controversy over whether the smallpox virus should be allowed to survive in "high-security" laboratories or be destroyed definitively. In 1978 a laboratory infection caused the death of a photographer in Birmingham, England. In 1980 the virus was maintained by six laboratories located in different countries and later was limited even more.

It has been argued that there should be no objection to the extinction, even in laboratories, of any virus that poses such a threat to people, whereas many species of harmless birds, fish, and mammals are eliminated without a thought. The other side of the argument has to do with the need for a reference sample of the true smallpox virus (*variola*). Scientists occasionally encounter other viruses of the "pox" family that pose no threat to humans. The only way to differentiate these variants from the *variola* strain is by comparing their individual DNA components. Human achievement, it seems, often leads to unforeseen problems. Who could have thought during the height of a smallpox epidemic that the day would come when people would advocate the controlled survival of the deadly virus?

Medicine can rightfully claim complete success in the fight against smallpox and polio, but even these spectacular accomplishments cannot entirely preclude the difficulties inherent in all immunization programs. Public apathy, physicians' skepticism, and too often misleading information detract from the benefits. Additionally, the emergence of a new epidemic, such as AIDS, may leave humankind without a remedy or prevention while scientists search for a solution.

Avoiding disease is superior to fighting it, even if the defense is as sophisticated a method as vaccination. Taking medication, getting injections, or staying on diets means effort, expense, and loss of time, the result being potential noncompliance. Measures that eliminate causes or risks are generally the most convenient and are eventually accepted as the least-disliked prescriptions that preventive medicine can give us.

Much of this work is done for us by public health agents, who inspect our food and water supply, exterminate mosquitoes, and perform a host of other life-saving tasks, as long as we make the needed funds available. Absolute prevention calls for an ever-increasing degree of control by governmental agencies in industry, commerce, agriculture, and pharmaceutics. The practical application of new knowledge creates new risks, and the public expects the authorities to take steps against anything that might make people sick.

This responsibility of the government is the subject of ongoing criticism. "Too little," "foot-dragging," "excessive," and "premature" are some of the frequent comments. Standards of occupational safety are often called unnecessary or restrictive, but should harm come to any employee from exposure to chemicals or radiation, the precautions are termed inadequate.

One of these necessary incursions by the government is the authority it exerts over the release of new drugs. The federal Food and Drug Administration (FDA) has established strict rules with which manufacturers must comply. Before the FDA will authorize the sale of a new drug, it may require a lengthy period of examination, which can be extremely costly to the manufacturer. Bureaucracy in action? Yes! But if we want to do justice to the FDA, we must not forget that the agency held up the release of thalidomide, thus sparing newborn infants in the United States that drug's disastrous effects. A regulatory agency like the FDA must have a resistance against risk-taking, preferring to have fewer drugs that are effective and safe rather than to release drugs that are effective but possibly unsafe. In an emergency (e.g., the appearance of a deadly and contagious disease such as AIDS), new drugs may be released early on a conditional basis.

Demands for much stronger governmental action have been voiced, particularly with regard to the prevention of cancer. Among these is a call for greater vigilance by already existing government agencies, such as the Environmental Protection Agency (EPA), the FDA, and the Occupational Safety and Health Administration (OSHA). New, powerful agencies specifically devoted to the fight against cancer have been suggested as well.

Our knowledge of the cause or causes responsible for the large number of cancer victims is fragmentary. It may seem logical, therefore, to indict all environmental risks for which a statistically significant association with malignant disease is recognized. Cancer has been called a disease of human origin. If this were true, the prevention of cancer would be within our reach.

Artificially produced evils are a matter for authoritative intervention. The government, backed by a strong national policy and proper legislation, can interdict all activities that might cause exposure of the public to cancer-related risks. Widening of the regulatory authority over pollution, food additives, drugs, and occupational hazards is in progress and is likely to accelerate steadily in the coming years. This will lead to more responsibility being given to agencies that design preventive measures and enforce them. It will require labor, funding, and above all, ready acceptance by those who are told what they must do or what they cannot do.

There is evidence, however, that the prevention of cancer may enter an entirely new field through the exploration of the genome. Research has identified a number of oncogenes, which may be regarded as mutant genes that either favor the development of malignant disease or fail to suppress it by replacing the normal suppressor genes. Prevention of cancer could eventually be based on the avoidance of external causes that lead to mutations and the formation of oncogenes.

With so much emphasis on exterminating parasites, killing bacteria, and banning cancer risks, one might think that we can prevent disease only by exclusion or destruction of causative agents. For some conditions, however, prophylaxis requires a positive approach based on the introduction of certain substances into the body.

The concept of the biological unit is based on the uninterrupted exchange of matter. The need for food and water is common knowledge, and their sustained lack is known to be incompatible with life. Requirements for other substances are less obvious, and awareness of them is in the territory of science. Research in this field has identified a number of conditions, notably the lack of vitamins, that can be forestalled or cured only by supplying the missing substance. An early example of this principle was the use of citrus juice against scurvy, introduced by naval surgeon James Lind in the late 1700s.

Diseases caused by the lack of some vital component are not as much in the mind of the public as conditions that are induced by infection, poisons, radiation, or any other external agent. Specific defects, often congenital, nevertheless occupy many pages in medical textbooks, and the victims can often be protected from serious damage. Hemophiliacs, for example, lack a clotting factor in their blood. This substance can be supplied, thus preventing their death from blood loss when they have a bleeding episode or must undergo surgery. Cretinism should become a condition of only historical interest if newborns are tested promptly for thyroid deficiency, which can be corrected by appropriate medication.

Our knowledge of conditions caused by deficiencies of vitamins, such as scurvy, rickets, and pellagra, suggests that the lack of other substances may be responsible for ailments of obscure origins. It is consequently tempting to believe that the daily intake of easily supplied preparations might be a simple means of prevention.

A conscientious investigator will be reluctant to encourage the daily use of any substance until it has stood the test of time, even if he or she is personally convinced of its value and safety. The daily use of aspirin for the prevention of strokes has been the subject of long-term research. The noted neurologist Dr. William Fields told a reporter, "You're talking to a man who takes one tablet twice a day and has for ten years. But I don't feel that, in good conscience, I could recommend that for everyone. What I do for myself is at my own personal risk."[12]

Such personal risk is typical of our preventive efforts. The experts cannot assure us that aspirin is efficient for the prevention of strokes and without potential danger. Nonetheless, millions will continue the aspirin prophylaxis as their free choice and at their own risk. The future will tell—perhaps! In the meantime, aspirin has been beneficial to the victims of heart attacks by reducing the incidence of second attacks.

Whereas the aspirin project aims at the prevention of a specific disease, other efforts are of a more general nature and emphasize life-style instead of medication. The scope of health movements tends to become wider as people receive information through books, lectures, and the news media. The roles of nutrition, environment, stress, and exercise are shown to be important for health, as are the emotional and religious aspects of life. The desire for a total approach finds expression in the holistic health movement, which sees the human mind and body as a system capable of warding off disease. This concept involves no unified theory, nor does it represent a special field of the practice of medicine.

It has been pointed out that a patient would have to make many office visits if the holistic approach were entirely the responsibility of physicians, but most facets of this trend concern matters that each person must weigh and decide for him- or herself. Some of its aspects are speculative, and many await proof by prolonged trial and unbiased analysis. This can be said also of the new medications and technical methods that physicians employ, however, and it should not discredit the holistic idea. The very fact that the individual is personally involved is in its favor. It is not limited to the sick trying to get well but applies particularly to those who want to stay in good health. Its most appealing feature is the emphasis on prevention of disease through modification in our daily living.

Any solidly established institution, regardless of how long its tradition or how brilliant its record, must be receptive to new ideas if it is to survive. It must be able to accept reasonable criticism and, at the same time, reject any unjustified accusations. Medicine as it is presently taught and practiced has become the subject of severe criticism. The critics tell us that, near the end of the twentieth century, medicine still relies on nineteenth-century concepts and is treating disease instead of preserving health.

Control of worms, mosquitoes, fleas, viruses, and bacteria is taken for granted now, and few of us bother to think about how much of our health this control preserves every day. Yet preventive medicine surely is not confined to parasitology, bacteriology, or virology. On the contrary, a vast number of prophylactic techniques have been introduced in the last few decades, based mainly on discoveries in biochemistry and immunology.

An example of this progress is the prophylaxis for hemolytic disease of the newborn. Detection of Rh incompatibility is an important part of prenatal care. Although affected infants can be treated with transfusions of compatible blood, the need for treatment has declined markedly since the 1960s, when researchers developed a preventive method based on the suppression of the mother's immune response. Injection of Rh-immuno-globulin (Rhogam) within three days after delivery inhibits the forma-tion of antibodies in the mother and removes the hazard to the next baby.[13] This injection has to be repeated near the end of each pregnancy and af-ter any miscarriage.

The suppression of the mother's immune response means that she is treated to protect the infant of the next pregnancy. Without antibodies there is no chance of hemolytic disease in the newborn. Absolute preven-tion is accomplished even before the baby is conceived. This type of pro-phylaxis goes beyond anything that preventive medicine offered in the past. Medical science has thus taken a near-perfect step in the direction of a disease-free state. The only flaw, however slight, is the need for an injection that can be inadvertently omitted through error or after an unrecognized miscarriage. In addition, Rh-positive blood from a trans-fusion occasionally may sensitize an Rh-negative woman. She will then have antibodies that are potentially harmful to an Rh-positive infant of any future pregnancy.

Complete circumvention of the Rh problem through selection of Rh-compatible parents is possible. *Theoretically,* it would be superior to the injection of immunoglobulin, but no one could seriously suggest that wedding plans be canceled when a near-perfect preventive method is available for solving such a problem.

The majority of the genetic diseases can be controlled only by prevent-ing the birth of an affected child. Genetic counseling has much to offer to prospective parents. It can tell them about their chances of having a normal child or about the kind of abnormality that might appear in their offspring. It is possible, for instance, to detect some serious hereditary disorders early in fetal life.

The main tool for prenatal diagnosis is amniocentesis. It is usually done around the sixteenth week of gestation, at which time a sample of the amniotic fluid is obtained through a puncture of the mother's abdomi-nal wall and the womb. The sample contains body cells of the fetus together with blood cells and chemical constituents. When grown in a tissue culture, the cells are suitable for an analysis of their chromosomes. This may reveal serious genetic disorders, notably Down's syndrome, which is a common cause of mental retardation.

Biochemical examination of the fluid or of the cultured cells can detect inborn errors of metabolism as well. These are mainly defects of vital enzymes leading to abnormal storage of lipids, carbohydrates, or amino acids in the fetal tissues. Congenital defects of the central nervous system, particularly anencephaly (absence of the brain) and spina bifida (incomplete closure of the spinal canal) are often associated with elevated levels of a specific substance (alpha-feto-protein) in the amniotic fluid. The concentration of this substance is also frequently elevated in the mother's blood.[14]

Certain risk categories warrant amniocentesis. One of these risk factors is a maternal age of thirty-five years or over. Research has shown that the incidence of Down's syndrome in infants born to mothers in this age group is significantly increased. Other indications for fetal chromosome analysis are a history of a previous child with a chromosome abnormality, multiple congenital anomalies in previous offspring, and certain chromosomal deviations of the parents. An alternative method to amniocentesis is the biopsy of the placenta (chorionic villus biopsy), which can be performed at an earlier stage of pregnancy.[15]

The condition of the fetus can be explored further through fetal visualization. Ultrasound, requiring no ionizing radiation, is the primary tool and can detect hydrocephalus and many other abnormalities.

Aside from making an intrauterine diagnosis, geneticists can detect carrier states of many hereditary disorders. Members of families in which such conditions have appeared are candidates for screening. In the case of some abnormalities for which groups have a relatively high incidence, carrier screening enables individuals to appraise their risk status. For example, being black or Jewish puts one in a higher risk category for sickle-cell anemia or Tay-Sachs disease, respectively. Both conditions are autosomal recessive disorders. Carriers are free of the disease, although specific tests may reveal their ability to transmit the condition to their offspring. This is the case in persons with the sickle-cell trait, which is present in carriers of sickle-cell anemia and can be identified by a simple screening method.

Genetic medicine has greatly increased in importance during the past few decades, but although the tools for detection are available, prevention of genetic diseases is still limited to a few options, none of which is entirely satisfactory from the human point of view.[16] Within the limits of legal and religious considerations, the family can elect to terminate the pregnancy. Experts on genetic counseling are quick to emphasize that this alternative must be considered on an individual basis and that such decisions must take into account the parents' beliefs.

New technology is rapidly expanding the realm of genetic counseling. It has been found that embryos may remain viable after long periods of freezing and may subsequently be implanted in the uterus. These preserved embryos can be screened, and the parents can make selections according to their wishes by rejecting those that they consider undesirable. It is debatable, at best, whether this selection can stand the scrutiny of medical, ethical, or legal considerations.

There is already a clandestine tendency among some parents to determine the sex of the fetus. They may then opt for an abortion if the unborn child is not of the desired sex. This tendency should be unacceptable to society, if only for the reason that the selection may upset the balance of nature and have consequences that we cannot possibly foresee. Prenatal selection is treading on dangerous ground and calls for prudence and caution rather than uncritical acceptance.

The discovery of the structure of DNA has advanced our knowledge to a point where experts can alter genes. We have received a tool of unbelievable potential, and researchers plan to use it on bacteria, plants, and animals—including humans. We are asking ourselves whether a modification of the human genetic code is feasible. If it were possible, would it also be safe and compatible with legal, moral, and religious concepts? Will DNA manipulation have a place in our quest for a disease-free state?

It is tempting to think that one could make subtle changes within the DNA molecule and thereby eliminate genetic characteristics that are conducive to disease. Mutant genes might be converted back to their normal antecedents. Scientists can already cut DNA into fragments and reassemble them to produce recombinant (spliced) DNA. This method is the basis for supplying cells with new genes that enable them to perform new functions. Science can thus produce bacteria that make needed substances such as insulin, or it can furnish industry with bacteria for mopping up oil spills. There have not yet been any significant safety problems with the new technology.

Qualified specialists, as well as the general public, have been understandably resistant to any suggestions of gene engineering in humans. The long-term effects of this technique are still unknown and could be devastating. The threat of disaster, however, seems remote if we do not manipulate the sex cells but deal only with the genes of the body cells (autosomal genes). We can use cells from a healthy person as a graft to replace the patient's defective genes, as long as the graft is compatible with the host. This method has met with some success through transplants of bone marrow in a variety of diseases including some types of anemias and in the severe combined immunodeficiency disease (SCID). The latter is a congenital disorder that is often fatal in the first year of life.

When we speak of altering the genetic code, however, we refer to the genes of the sex cells rather than the autosomal genes. This means tampering with the genetic material that will be transmitted from one generation to another. Before we take this fateful step, we must be aware that it could unleash catastrophic events beyond our control.

It is obvious that we must await clearance from the most qualified specialists in the fields of genetic engineering, law, and ethics before we can regard this new branch of science as possibly applicable to humans. While we are waiting, we might speculate about a related problem. Could genetic engineering of humans fulfill our dream of attaining the disease-free state? The logical reply is that this seems unlikely. Any remodeling of our genetic code would be based on our current concept of what is best for us. Whenever we act to improve our lot, we are likely to encounter unexpected complications. We might change human genetic structure to our advantage, but we cannot foresee the nature of future risks and cannot build protection against them into any new genetic code. We would still fail to react properly to environmental challenges of our own making that will result in disease.

The record of preventive medicine is impressive, and it deserves our confidence. The history of vaccination, from Jenner to Salk and Sabin, is cause for hope of future achievements, as is the enormous reduction in the mortality from epidemics. Even limited prevention, which detects and treats subclinical disease, represents great progress.

At present we hope for more absolute prevention through avoidance of known risks, but this approach requires a constant expansion of public health measures. These bring new restrictions and obligations not only for the big corporate manufacturers but also for the workers, farmers, food processors, and many others. We might simply say that new controls affect the entire populace, since all of us are potential violators of environmental safety.

Our wishful thoughts of the disease-free state are like our dreams of permanent peace. They ignore human nature and the essence of life. Neither is compatible with a secure existence but calls for frequent change and risk taking. Absolute prevention is the ideal way of eradicating disease. It has great merits when we are dealing with parasites, microbes, or other natural causes, but we find that we often cannot avoid the risks that we ourselves create.

We can see a gradual development in the history of medicine. At first, there were attempts to cure or alleviate physical suffering. Then came practical methods of prevention—first, for children and adults; later, for the fetus; and finally, for the life that is yet to begin. Modern-day health care must consider future generations, although few methods that might serve this purpose are available at present. There is much public concern about this phase of medical protection, particularly about the ban of any physical or chemical agent that might cause mutations.

The human-made alterations of the environment began long ago through uncontrolled pollution by smoke and wastes. Until recently these infractions were small in number, and their impact was almost negligible. The twentieth century brought a dramatic escalation of uncritical tampering with the environment, but it also saw the beginning of our awareness. The future will see greater control through avoidance or active manipulation of risk factors.

We are engaged in competition for the means of existence. Our competitors are humans and the other creatures of the earth—and possibly extraterrestrial beings in the future. To compete we rely on technology as our principal weapon. Its by-products are risk factors that constantly change and therefore are not amenable to absolute prevention. Our best defense against these unplanned creations of our inventive minds is watchfulness, leading to early detection of trouble and, subsequently, to immediate intervention. This approach will not lead us to the utopian land where there is no disease, but it will at least ensure that we travel in the right direction.

8

The Human Reaction

Medicine is as old as human society, and man has
always attempted to understand and deal with
disease in the same terms in which he attempts to
understand himself and his creations.

—Leland J. Rather, Preface to *Selected
Essays of Rudolf Virchow*

The impact of disease on society is
determined by the attitude of the individual, for no health project can succeed unless it is supported by the majority of the people who are supposed
to benefit from it. When we consider the type of disease that has clinical
manifestations, the question of its impact is easily answered. Pain, discomfort, and inactivity are by and large unacceptable to anyone. Ascetic training, self-discipline, or hypnosis may modify the feeling of a few victims,
but their number is negligible. In general, the human reaction to any
evidence of disease is one of distress, fear, and often horror or despair.

The desire to obtain immediate relief is the obvious reaction to any
awareness of disease. Victims seek medical treatment that they expect to
end the pain and restore normal conditions. They desire as well release
from the threat of death that is associated with disease.

Our attitude toward manifest disease can therefore be characterized as our search for a cure that will terminate the intrusion on our physical comfort. In fact, we often equate medical attention with cure, thinking that any ailment yields to a specific treatment, usually a drug, sometimes hot packs or cold packs, or occasionally surgery.

The average patient's image of medicine is confined mainly to alleviating and curative activities. The approach is positive and reasonably optimistic. The person trusts the members of the medical profession but sometimes prefers self-proclaimed healers who have had no regular training. This preference tends to go hand-in-hand with uncritical acceptance of hearsay information regarding wonder drugs.

The average person's resistance to thoughts of "being sick without knowing it" is actually a sane and purposeful reaction. It protects us from undue concern over potential sickness and prevents excessive expenditure of time and money for medical attention. If we think of our state of health as a fluid condition rather than a static one, we understand that variations of this state occur constantly and are counteracted by adjustments. Reliance on our ability to compensate for most disruptions of our physical balance is a prerequisite to being reasonably well adjusted.

The spirit of private enterprise entails a sense of responsibility for one's health. Each person is expected to look after his or her own well-being by dieting, regular checkups, exercise, and other measures that are currently advocated. The implication is that we will have to blame ourselves if we neglect our bodies and become sick. The same mandates that govern our material possessions are applied to our physical condition. Put up a fight! Conquer disease! Be in control!

This rigid attitude may guarantee success in business or sports, but it has limitations in biology. Psychologists have pointed out that we must recognize the limits of our power over ourselves and that the notion of omnipotence is inapplicable to health care. We do have control over some hazards to our health, but these constitute only a fraction of the potential threats to our well-being.

The desire to act efficiently and thereby ensure success is rooted in the tradition of the Western world. The Western spirit cherishes the do-it-yourself principle and believes that there is a practical way to any goal. Lack of success implies personal failure and evokes a sense of inadequacy. This mentality might make victims of an illness feel that they should have prevented it and that they brought it on themselves through neglect.

Contemporary thinking emphasizes individual responsibility for nearly everything. Existentialism as expressed by Jean-Paul Sartre sees war and other great calamities as the results of decisions in which each of the victims had a choice. He explains, "Man being condemned to be free carries the weight of the whole world on his shoulders; he is responsible for the world and for himself as a way of being." And he concludes, "We have the war we deserve."[1] If we accept this line of reasoning, we may add that we have the *disease* we deserve.

Older schools of thought, particularly Buddhism and other Eastern philosophies, teach acceptance of illness and death. They stress the individual's submission to the vastness of nature. According to this view, disease is part of life. We have no authority over it and must yield when it strikes. Unconditional acceptance of ill health has no place in the world of the twentieth century, however, except in obedience to special religious dogmas. The most powerful rhetoric could not persuade a significant number of citizens of any country to tolerate pain without seeking help or to reject preventive measures of proven value. If we fall ill through self-neglect, be it willful or born of ignorance, we have indeed the illness we deserve.

When illness strikes and we realize that no cure is at hand, we need the spirit of the Stoics:

> What does bearing a fever rightly mean? It means not to blame God or man, not to be crushed by what happens, to await death in a right spirit, to do what you are bidden.[2]

> The pain which is intolerable carries us off; but that which lasts a long time is tolerable, and the mind maintains its own tranquility by retiring into itself.[3]

The time for action, however, is before we fall victim to disease, when we think ahead in the spirit of self-reliance, responsibility, and determination. Hegel writes, "I am free, when my existence depends upon myself."[4] Schopenhauer declares, "As the human body generally corresponds to the human will, so the individual body structure corresponds to the individually modified will, the character of the individual."[5]

Responsibility in a wider sense implies progress through collective support of research and public health measures, for whatever care the individual receives depends on the availability of competent medical personnel and adequate facilities. By ignoring the medical needs of the community, the nation, or the world, we open the door to the illness that we deserve.

When we assume the responsibility for our own well-being, we must understand that this does not give us control over the hazards to our health. People may be fully aware of all their obligations and live up to them as well as they can and yet be sick during their entire lives. This discrepancy stems from the gap that lies between the extent of human achievement and the magnitude of adversities still to be overcome. The gap is present not only in the health field but in practically every aspect of human existence.

We try to regulate behavior within our society by law, but although humankind has made laws since time immemorial and has devised institutions to interpret and enforce them, crime is rampant throughout the world. We have harnessed the oil and minerals of the earth and even learned how to split the atom, yet we are facing an energy crisis. Neither the automobile, the airplane, nor the space rocket has brought us an adequate solution to our transportation problems. Similarly, after wiping out smallpox and learning to control poliomyelitis, we are still helpless against a host of other viral diseases.

Humankind recognizes and accepts the obligation to improve its lot. "I know of no more encouraging fact," says Henry Thoreau in *Walden,* "than the unquestionable ability of man to elevate his life by a conscious endeavor."[6] In all fields of endeavor the pattern is the same. Any generation has individuals with a strong urge to help society advance. Some of them succeed in making great discoveries or inventions, but this progress is but a fraction of an inch on a road that has no end.

On our side of the gap is the sum of human accomplishments. They include the defenses we have devised, the accumulated medical knowledge that we use to assist and complement the natural defense mechanism of the body. This conquered ground is pitifully small if compared with what lies on the other side of the gap, where perils against which we have no adequate remedies form an endless line stretching toward the horizon. Anyone contemplating that line must know that our control is greatly limited in scope and that we cannot hope to prevent or cure all our potential ills.

Failure to realize our limitations will doom us to disappointment and make us easy prey to unfounded claims by would-be healers. It creates an atmosphere of tension and insecurity. Regardless of what we are doing for our health, there always remains some measure we have not tried that might guarantee disease-free survival to a ripe age. Awareness of this leads to guilt feelings in persons who fall ill and believe that they could have remained well if only they had eaten pure natural food, taken more vitamins, or gone for more checkups. Finally, this illusion of unlimited control causes an unwarranted ballooning of the health industry, with escalation of expenses and excessive demands on personnel.

Like all creatures, humans have the ability to adjust to adversity, to compensate for loss of function, and to repair damage. When disease strikes, these properties are invaluable aids for surviving periods of distress and disability. Unlike the animals, however, we can analyze the ills that befall us and devise methods to overcome them. We rely principally on our power to act rationally instead of on physical strength, swift flight, or camouflage.

The need for passive as well as active resistance exceeds the teachings of any single philosopher. The readiness to endure suffering is only our last choice. It is unthinkable as a permanent attitude that would let disease have its course. That we must accept death does not mean we need accept pain or other forms of physical distress, for we have the inborn desire, as well as sometimes the ability, to improve the conditions of our lives. The spirit of self-reliance, responsibility, and determination gives constant impetus to the human-made phase of our resistance to disease.

Human beings deal with the fluctuations of physical conditions in a most complex way. While the disturbance is still below the threshold of our awareness, we automatically initiate defenses against it. When this resistance fails, we retreat, cut our losses, and adjust to our new position.

Awareness comes when painful sensations begin or when experience tells us that danger exists without causing distress at the moment. In either case we have to decide whether we should seek professional help, wait, or act on our own. Each decision has its own problems. To whom should we turn for help? How will we make the necessary arrangements for compensation and loss of time? By what measures can we prevent similar disruptions of our activities in the future?

We are at all times confronted with the necessity of making choices, and those choices affect our future. Tomorrow's events always carry the stamp of the decisions we make today. But they are also shaped by developments that we cannot control. In the case of disease, our inability to control it is in a way a product of our decisions, for it represents the human-made phase of our defense, which we can either promote through active support or retard through lack of interest.

Humankind moves from one generation to the next in a perpetual quest for the domination of disease. The aging of our bodies is a process that we must learn to endure, yet we want to prevent and combat the ills that accompany it as best we can.

The bodies of humans and animals are superbly equipped to cope with the world outside them. The inner balance of any organism is maintained by innumerable devices that make adjustments to any change of environment and adapt to it as far as possible. If necessary, they can initiate repair of injury and restoration of normal conditions. In some instances the offending cause can be eliminated, as a thorn is extracted from the skin, or there may be immediate recoil after contact with the injurious agent, as when one accidentally touches a flame. This tendency to safeguard the inner balance depends on functions that need no conscious effort. They are set in motion by impulses traveling through the nervous system and are mediated by the action of hormones.

The automatic reaction to external agents is common to humans and animals alike. Humans, however, possess another system of defense that is the product of their own planning and designing. The development of the human brain allows the coordination of observed facts or events. It makes it possible, furthermore, to draw conclusions and to use them for practical applications. This ability is the basis for our conscious effort to resist any disturbance of our internal balance. The human-made defense ordinarily goes into action when the individual is aware of deviations from the normal condition; in its most accomplished form, however, it enables us to anticipate and prevent potential threats to our well-being.

Humankind's way of safeguarding health is much the same as its approach to technical problems. By combining experience with observation and intuition, we assist our built-in defense mechanisms and thereby restore our internal balance. Bacteria are checked with penicillin or other antibiotics, cancerous tissues are excised, and lost blood cells are replaced by transfusion. Vaccination stimulates the production of antibodies that may have been absent. Hormones that normally mediate the body's response to stress can be supplied as medication if their natural action is inadequate. Drugs extracted from plants and animal tissue, or made synthetically, are available to kill pain, regulate the heart beat, control blood pressure, and perform many other desirable tasks.

By using their unique abilities, human beings have immensely complicated the interplay between the individual and the surrounding world. High-speed vehicles, a classic example of human ingenuity, increase the number and seriousness of accidental injuries and cause respiratory disease through air pollution. New methods of prevention and medical treatment must therefore be devised to deal with the adverse effects of the internal combustion engine and the powerful conveyances that it has made possible. The corrective measures may minimize the adverse effects of the engine but cannot eliminate them entirely. The diverse applications of this device, represented most prominently by the automobile, belong to the progress of civilization; they give humans a useful tool that they will not relinquish until a better one is available. With the new convenience have come new external perils, both physical and chemical, that will cause disease unless we can cope with them.

The example of the internal combustion engine illustrates a pattern that recurs with any great technical invention. The development of atomic energy may present problems of greater magnitude, but the principle that applied to the splitting of the atom holds true for the introduction of the automobile. We are acquiring a new source of power at the cost of certain threats to our physical well-being. The foremost risk is exposure to radiation, which has immediate effects in the form of radiation sickness. Delayed consequences of radiation are leukemia, cancer, and malformations of the newborn.

In spite of controversy and protests, it is safe to predict that we will accept the risks inherent in the use of nuclear energy and will try to minimize them by preventive methods. Should these fail, the victims will receive medical treatment that may be grossly inadequate at first but will surely become more efficient in response to the growing need.

Humankind's propensity for assuming risks is not fundamentally different from the behavior of animals that leave the safety of their lairs in search of food and expose themselves to predators. The difference lies in the conscious design of potentially harmful devices and activities in the course of human progress. In addition to facing naturally existing dangers, humans must constantly meet new challenges that are of their own making.

Suffering, or fear of suffering, causes people to accept any offer of relief, often without first examining it. The threat of disease is ever present, and with it goes the wish to escape by whatever means might seem promising. Unproved remedies are eagerly accepted by the sick; commercially advertised preventive drugs have a lucrative market among customers who demand no record of proven performance. Alexander of Tralles wrote in the sixth century, "For epilepsy take a nail of a wrecked ship, make it into a bracelet and set therein the bone of a stag's heart taken from its body whilst alive; put it on the left arm; you will be astonished at the result."[7]

The following twentieth-century newspaper headline suggests similar gullibility: "Top Doctor Says Simple Addition to Diet Will Cut Cancer by 80–90 Percent."[8]

This uncritical acceptance finds its greatest potential in the field of nutrition.[9] Any person armed simply with the knowledge of a high school graduate must know that it requires controlled research to confirm any alleged cause-and-effect relation (see chap. 4). Nevertheless, the same person will pay good money for an item of health food recommended to protect against colds and to maintain sexual potency. Ruth Gay writes in "Fear of Food," "Although we learned long ago to abandon magical thinking in connection with weather, crops, the care of animals and other natural phenomena, it still has us in its grip when we think of our diet. Our latest thinking about food, based on fear, is proportionately retrograde— willing to accept, indeed seeking out, the consolation of magic, the mute practices of peasants and the quaint devices of folklore."[10]

Imagination and desire are often substitutes for facts: "wishing will make it so." This is particularly relevant for persons who have contracted a disease. Any illness affects the mind and makes it more susceptible to suggestion. It is easy to reason that nothing is impossible and that others have lived after they had been given up by the doctors. Magic supersedes facts and reason.

Fad diets and wonder drugs find their victims not only among the sick but also among healthy persons, whom they tempt with hopes of better and lasting health. Anything that is thoroughly advertised can be made believable. People who follow the same fad are a group of believers, perfecting a cult that gives them pride and confidence. The proud statement "We eat only natural food" implies that only the ignorant masses disregard this rule and contaminate themselves with unnatural food that is presumedly tainted by chemicals.

If advertised claims were subject to the same scrutiny that is applied to potential causes of cancer, the process, although time-consuming and expensive, would save countless people from wasting their money on worthless miracle drugs, health foods, and books on simple ways to health. When accepting health measures that have not been tested by approved methods, we throw away our ability to discriminate and to choose after examining. The expected benefit may be illusionary, or the effect may actually be harmful. The way of the animals acting on instinct is surely preferable to that of the health faddists yielding to the enticement of commercial advertising.

The tendency to submit to health fads is fortunately only one aspect of human nature. More important is the rational desire to fight disease by proven methods. Any creature possesses automatic mechanisms that attempt to maintain or restore its biological balance. These functions are a part of the genetic code. They are furnished "free" by nature. The extragenetic faculties are peculiar to humans. They are the products of knowledge that is either newly acquired or has been handed from one generation to the next.

Human beings rely greatly on their extragenetic heritage. We take it for granted that there is a key to every secret and a cure for every ill because uncounted generations have made contributions to the knowledge on which we depend. Our rationally based activities in the medical arena deal mainly with the noticeable manifestations of disease. They are intended to alleviate pain or abolish it and to restore usefulness. The cure is the supreme achievement of the human contribution. To cure an ill, however, means that the ill is first allowed to come into existence. Since disease is a signal of biological imbalance, the concept of the cure implies that we let balance be lost and then alleviate the effect of the imbalance. We repair the roof instead of protecting it from damage.

Medicine has not neglected the prevention of disease, however. The incidence of epidemics has been reduced through vaccination and public health measures, and some diseases have ceased to exist in their epidemic form. We do not usually honor these accomplishments as much as we marvel at new drugs or surgical operations. The persons who kept a war from breaking out tend to remain obscure, whereas victorious generals are recorded in the annals of history.

In spite of the feats of preventive medicine, we look to medicine mainly for cures by surgery or medication. Prevention means forethought, and most people find it inconvenient to think ahead. There is always the expectation that relief is available on request when necessary. It is tempting to speculate on the relation of preventive thought to a wait-and-see attitude. Could it be that a preventive attitude requires a higher level of intelligence than one geared to immediate action? Is *Homo sapiens* gradually moving upward into an intellectual atmosphere where forethought is prevalent?

If this assumption is correct, we nevertheless find that at the end of the twentieth century the average individual is still very much a creature of the present, living his or her own life and giving little thought to the welfare of future generations. National politics, economy, and international diplomacy reflect day-to-day decisions rather than long-term planning. As John Dewey wrote in *Human Nature and Conduct,* "The present, not the future, is ours. No shrewdness, no store of information will make it ours."[11]

Scientists and technologists have been ahead of politicians and financiers in the human movement toward foresight. Visions of air travel, atom splitting, and conquest of outer space were methodically brought to fruition. Plans to control disease through sanitary measures or immunizations have been faithfully followed for decades, and systematic elimination of cancer risk factors will benefit future generations.

Still, the present generation demands the full attention of the medical profession, and it wants to receive immediate benefits. Its expectations of the human contribution to the fight against disease are limitless. There must be a pill or an operation for any complaint.

After an injury, such as a laceration of the skin, our genetically conferred reactions go into effect automatically. The damaged nerves cause pain. Blood vessels contract to minimize blood loss, and leukocytes aggregate to fight bacteria. An injured person who then seeks medical attention thereby enters the extragenetic phase of reaction to the injury. Depending on the extent of the damage, the artificial defense may consist of a simple surgical suture, or it may require hospitalization, antibiotics, and blood transfusions.

All these measures depend on organized facilities that are the products of long-term research and planning. A blood transfusion, for instance, must be preceded by recruitment of suitable donors and the drawing and storage of blood, which require trained personnel to perform blood typing, crossmatching, and other tests that guarantee the safety of the procedure. Additional personnel are needed to administer the transfusion and to monitor it.

No matter how advanced and sophisticated the technical accomplishments may seem to us, the extragenetic phase has none of the smooth perfection that characterizes the body's own reaction to injury. Medical care is predicated on the judgment of individuals and is therefore subject to human error. Its availability requires constant businesslike preparations, and it may be absent when needed.

Whereas the natural devices are silent and continuously regulated, the approach designed by humans is often confusing, piecemeal, and dependent on personal initiative. The human contribution could not succeed on its own, but when combined with the natural defenses, it may be decisive and life-saving. We call this combination a cure, a triumph over evil, a victory that puts an end to suffering.

The excision of an inflamed appendix is considered a cure. Unless complications arise, there will be an end to pain and fever and a return to health. The era of the antibiotics, beginning with Fleming's discovery of penicillin, has made cures of formidable diseases possible. Tuberculosis, meningitis, endocarditis, and pneumonia can be overcome without permanent damage. Even victims of dread epidemics such as plague and cholera can be saved.

The most sober reasoning cannot deny credit to medical science for its success in dealing decisively with individual ailments. The same process of reasoning, however, makes us realize that a cure, no matter how complete, is not the best way to safeguard our health. To be made well is inferior to being kept well. Besides, there are potential complications inherent in any form of treatment. When we are dealing with biological conditions, we cannot predict the course of events with certainty. No matter how far science may advance, life will always be ahead of it and come up with surprises that the most sophisticated calculations cannot anticipate.

These surprise developments may defeat the attempt of a cure or turn it into a separate illness. We do not know why one person in thousands suffers cardiac arrest while under anesthesia, or why some patients are sensitive to drugs that generally are well tolerated.

The ramifications of medical treatment are not confined to simple side reactions but may be exceedingly intricate and require thorough investigation before their true nature is recognized. Nosocomial (hospital-acquired) infections posed a threat in the 1950s and 1960s, when some particularly virulent strains of bacteria, notably *Staphylococcus aureus,* were rampant in hospitalized patients.[12] This development was explained by the resistance of these strains to antibiotics. Many patients in medical institutions were treated with antibiotics, and the resistant bacteria survived in enormous numbers in the wards and rooms. Disinfection and other hygienic measures were needed to protect patients and personnel from this hospital-borne hazard.

The problem of resistant strains was later overcome by new antibiotics, and nosocomial infections were minimized for a number of years. In recent times, however, this menace has returned, particularly for patients with tuberculosis (see chap. 7). It also complicates infections with other microorganisms.[13] The existence of these resistant strains illustrates how efforts at healing may spawn new diseases. This dilemma is typical of the atmosphere in which medicine must operate. It is a reflection of humankind's perpetual problem posed by the unexpected by-products of our progress. Insecticides kill pests but may also damage the body's vital enzyme systems. Life-saving drugs may bring iatrogenic diseases. Penicillin, for instance, can cause severe allergic reactions associated with fever and skin rash. In rare cases, potentially fatal shock may occur.

Adverse drug reactions are so numerous that it is virtually impossible to keep abreast of new information concerning them. We realize the magnitude of the problem when we read that in 1978, 2,000 incidents of drug-induced disease of the eye alone were reported to the FDA.

To minimize undesirable effects, or to enhance beneficial results, technical procedures must frequently be revised and become more involved. Therefore, services that are designed to alleviate specific conditions tend to proliferate. Modifications that represent only slight improvements may nevertheless call for new equipment and personnel, and consequently for greater expenditures.

Just such an increase is illustrated by a cost analysis of specific improvements in some medical procedures. In a study that combined medicine with biostatistics, Marc Rosenschein and his associates at the University of Washington examined the cost effectiveness of transfusing concentrates of white blood cells.[14] Patients receiving intensive chemotherapy for acute leukemia often suffer a marked reduction in the number of their white blood cells (leukocytes) and are highly susceptible to infections. Transfusions of leukocytes can prevent 50–75 percent of early deaths from infections. They would add approximately 10.9 percent to the hospital bill of the average leukemic patient and cost 17.7 million dollars annually nationwide. These figures apply only to *therapeutic* transfusions—those that are given when there is already evidence of infection. For *prophylactic* transfusions, given to leukemic patients before infection has set in, the figures are 35.2 percent per hospital bill and 57.8 million dollars annually. The financial information given in the study by Rosenschein may have changed, but the principle of his findings remains the same.

The example of the leukocyte transfusions helps us to understand the dilemma facing us when we pay attention to cost effectiveness. May we deny desperately sick persons any slight advantage we can give them, even if the expense is exorbitant? Does not society have to provide the means for making this treatment possible?

Since improved techniques are constantly introduced, we must expect an astronomical escalation of costs. The *Health Care Financing Review of 1979,* published by the Department of Health, Education and Welfare (now the Department of Health and Human Services), indicates that from 1968 to 1978 total yearly national health expenditures rose from 58.9 billion dollars to 192.4 billion. By 1980 we were already well above the 200 billion dollar mark.

As long as our fight against disease is mainly a matter of combating it after it has gained a foothold, we must be prepared to pay the costs in terms of suffering, disability, and money. We cannot afford to abandon this approach until methods of prevention gradually replace the methods of treatment. In the eubiotic state disease either cannot develop or it is detected and eliminated while still in its preclinical phase. We are in search of this state and moving toward it.

It is human nature to take pride in one's possessions. This tendency may have to be subdued when it becomes the excessive, unbridled materialistic desire to have and to hold. Opinions about the pride of possessing run the gamut from contempt to praise in literature and philosophy. When it comes to interest in the state of our health, however, there is little argument, if any. It may be said that we do not own our bodies, but we at least have them on loan during our lifetimes. To care for this temporary possession should be proper in anyone's view.

The degree and the kind of care we want to use is subject to individual decision. An overanxious, hypochondriac tendency is as bad as a neglectful attitude. We have the assistance of the experts at our disposal. How much—or how little—use we make of it is a matter for personal decision. Nobody, expert or layperson, has all of the answers, and we find ourselves often in scientific terra incognita. How we make our way through this gray zone is the real test of our self-reliance.

9

Dialogue of the Ages

Time present and time past
Are both perhaps present in time future
And time future contained in time past.

—Thomas Stearns Eliot, *Four Quartets*

What is the future of medicine? Precisely what may we expect in the way of cure and prevention in the year 2500 or 3000? The writer of science fiction is free to paint a picture in vivid colors, describing the replacement of diseased organs, the eradication of bacteria, and the selective destruction of cancerous tissue. An imaginative mind can even posit new drugs that easily rejuvenate the body and double or triple the average life span.

Serious writers of science fiction base their predictions on facts and on the rules of probability. These authors may be posthumously justified by events that confirm what they had anticipated. Good science fiction is believable because it projects developments of discoveries or inventions that have already been made. Advances of the past few decades have brought us items that would have been interesting material for science fiction around the middle of the century. Predictions in physics and astronomy are likely to be more accurate than those in medicine, however, for medicine deals with biology and, more important perhaps, with human nature, which is unpredictable by our present scientific methods.

New developments in the health field are different from those of the exact sciences. Medical discoveries are often initiated by incidental observations rather than by logical reasoning. They also tend to become obsolete and are replaced by methods unrelated to them. In the 1930s there was a new cure for pneumonia based on a battery of antiserums, each of which was effective against a specific type of *pneumococcus*. It was a cumbersome procedure, requiring the typing of the *pneumococcus* before the specific serum could be selected. Nonetheless, the method was scientifically sound and proved effective. One might have anticipated that eventually there would be serums for most diseases caused by bacteria. The discovery of penicillin, coming a few years after the type-specific serum, provided a much simpler approach, and only a few infectious diseases are now treated with antiserum for quick, short effect.

Although it is futile and misleading to anticipate technical developments, predictions of a more general nature are justified if they rest on past experience and a knowledge of human behavior. The desire to improve our lot is inherent in our nature, and with it goes the determination to fight any forces that threaten our well-being. A few exceptional persons, through spiritual sublimation and ascetic self-control, may learn how to cope unaided with pain or disability. Their number is negligible, however, and in spite of their existence, it is clear that the vast majority will never accept physical distress willingly and will seek help to combat it.

Disease means the failure of the biological unit in its competition with other units. What will happen, in centuries to come, as the human units minimize their failures and become increasingly competitive? Our progress has placed us so far above most animals that their existence has become little more than a question of being tolerated. The fate of the animals is sealed, in spite of the valiant efforts of a few people to stem the tide. There does not seem to be enough room and food on the earth to accommodate all creatures. Whether or not they intend to do so, human beings are likely to exterminate fishes, amphibia, reptiles, birds, mammals, and perhaps themselves. But will they be superior in competing with insects, protozoa, bacteria, and viruses? We could be overrun by swarms of insecticide-immune gnats or invaded by bacteria resistant to antibiotics. Moreover, who can be sure that there are no living forms, smaller than viruses, of which we are not yet aware because our microscopes are not powerful enough to let us see them?

Changes in humankind's biological position have implications that go far beyond the territory of science. Questions of food, living space, and environment concern all people. Medical progress and the safety of medical procedures are of vital importance to society. News reporters, lawmakers, and administrators are instrumental, possibly more so than doctors, in shaping medical policy, and with this involvement comes the influence of politics.

Biological theories, particularly those of a general nature, are easily exploited for political ends. A favorite argument says that society has not only the right but the obligation to examine all products of research in science and make decisions for the common good. Society's wishes may be based on primitive beliefs, as was its ancient desire to be composed only of what it considered "normal" persons. This explains measures aimed at the control of the unfit that have ranged from legalized homicide of malformed infants in ancient times to twentieth-century laws for the sterilization of the mentally retarded. The concept of superior and poor blood lines became ingrained in popular thought through the centuries by the observations of animal breeders and by the acceptance of ruling dynasties believed to be the elite.

In 1859 Darwin published his thoughts under the title *The Origin of Species by Means of Natural Selection, or The Preservation of Favoured Races in the Struggle for Life.*[1] Near the end of this work we see the subtitle explained more fully: "In the preservation of favoured individuals and races, during the constantly recurrent struggle for Existence, we see the most powerful and ever-acting means of selection. The struggle for existence inevitably follows from the high geometrical ratio of increase which is common to all organic beings."[2] The Darwinian theory, so meticulously conceived and carefully documented, was nevertheless subjected to willful misinterpretation by a few to prove an inherited biological inferiority of certain individuals or ethnic groups.

From this distortion of science it was but one step to the generalization of the blood-and-race principle and its inclusion into a merciless national policy under the Nazi regime. What followed may be the greatest example of biology's penetration by politics, but it is not the only one. Under democratic freedom there is much nonmedical bickering over health issues. Controversies regarding recombinant DNA and atomic energy have profound medical implications and serve the propaganda aims of some group or another. The proposed ban on saccharin was argued in the Congress of the United States and then postponed repeatedly. Nothing is too technical or too insignificant to escape the political limelight.

All activities related to life have some territory in common and are bound to attract conflicting interests at times. Astronomy may be kept free of interference by the public or the public servants, but advances in biology are apt to affect everybody's life and become subject to public scrutiny. Medicine has depended to a great extent on the teaching of religion, ethics, and philosophy. Medicine can never be free of politics, for the politician must find ways to finance it, and with the money comes unavoidable control.

The care of our physical well-being, it seems, is inseparable from our general way of thought and from the conduct of our civic functions. When we try to formulate the ideal position of human society in the biological system, we soon realize that we are facing an insurmountable task. As denizens of the twentieth century, we are so far removed from the ideal situation that any attempt to describe it in today's setting would be ludicrous. To get an image of the perfect state of health preservation, we have to write socio-science fiction.

PLACE: all planets inhabited by humans
TIME: eons beyond A.D. 2000

Through the labors of uncounted scientists, society has at last realized that humans, like all other biological units, are fractions of the biological whole from which they are inseparable and on which they are totally dependent. The Governing Organization is aware of the following facts:

1. The flawless interplay of a unit with the whole results in the balanced state of the unit and in its optimal fitness for biological competition.
2. Any deviation from perfect interaction means disease. The magnitude of disease is determined by the equation $d = p - o$, where d is disease; p, the total of all disease-promoting factors; and o, the total of disease-opposing factors.
3. By applying this equation society has achieved complete biological balance and thereby reduced d to zero. This means that disease no longer exists in any form. It has been wiped out by a process of total prevention. To maintain our disease-free condition, the Governing Organization has issued the following rules, which regulate all phases of the life of each unit:

THESE HEALTH EDICTS PERTAIN, BUT ARE NOT LIMITED, TO BREATH-
ING, EATING, WORK, PLEASURE, SEX . . .

Science fiction. Utopia. We cannot attain it in the twentieth century,
nor do we want it at the price that the units of the story have to pay. Perhaps the enormous progress of science will bring with it a docile public
ready to let government regulate body functions. This transformation may
already have begun, but we are grateful for every inch that it has not yet
covered.

What general approach to health can we expect *today* and how much
government are we willing to accept for its sake? Surely the basic concept
of the futuristic tale is true. We *are* units of an immeasurable whole. Our
ability to interact smoothly with other parts of the whole determines our
state of health and our capacity for biological competition. Any deviation
from perfect interaction means disease.

Up to this point we have no cause to argue with the fiction writer. When
we come to the equation, however, we find that we cannot reduce d to zero.
Our knowledge of p and o is vastly inadequate for this problem, although
we work toward the solution. We strive for absolute prevention, meaning that we keep disease from developing instead of fighting it. Holistic
medicine tries to reach this goal with methods that affect all aspects of
life, such as psychological factors, nutrition, exercise, and environmental risks.

We get the impression that all these considerations have merits, but it
is most difficult, if not impossible, to formulate specific programs that are
practical and will stand the test of time. Taking only the question of diet,
we go from low-cholesterol to low-triglycerides and then back to low-
cholesterol, or better, low-fat—and possibly also to high-protein, high-
fiber, and high-vitamin.

Beneath the confusing evidence there is some commonsense truth that
remains valid even if the technical details become questionable. Caloric
limitations prevent overweight, which is unhealthy by anyone's standards.
Physical exercise, in some form, brings a sensation of well-being. Avoidance of psychological stress factors makes daily life easier, reduces emotional tension, and thereby lightens the burden on the heart and blood
vessels. Statistics persistently reflect less morbidity and relative longevity
for people who observe discipline in all their activities.

This evidence makes sense when applied to the concept of biological competition. How can one expect to be competitive by using pleasure as the only yardstick in deciding what to do and what not to do? The pleasure-seekers and lotus-eaters are quickly overcome by more disciplined contestants, much as liberal Athens succumbed to ascetic Sparta.

We have an obligation to adjust and control our life-styles according to the dictates of common sense. Unlike the human units of science fiction, we are not forced to observe prescribed rules. Instead, each person is responsible for formulating his or her own program. By using good judgment and obtaining professional advice, we should be able to choose wisely from the pool of scientific information.

We recognize that absolute prevention will not be perfected in our time and that it probably never will be. We consequently must cope with disease as best we can. Vaccination produces a minimal degree of disease sufficient to stimulate the production of antibodies. Recognition of subclinical conditions through detection programs enables us to put out the fire before it has caused serious harm. For a long time to come, however, we will still have to fight advanced disease with medication or surgery. The human-made phase of opposition to disease is likely to remain oriented toward the concept of a cure.

All these tasks have implications of a public nature. To think that activities as vital as health measures can be kept free of governmental involvement would be naïve. The most we can hope for is that in the future, biological science and medicine will not be used for political purposes as they sometimes have been in the past.

What is the ultimate aim of medical endeavor? Beyond the promise of an end to pain and the hope for a cure lies the faint image of the ideal eubiotic state from which disease is banished by human ingenuity. To approach this goal poses an ongoing challenge, a mandate handed from one generation to the next. In the eubiotic state disease is not allowed to gain a foothold. Humankind's own devices enhance or supplement the natural mechanism of defense: we strengthen resistance against viruses or microbes through vaccination; we use knowledge of potential hazards to avoid injury effectively; and exercise, diet, and medication give us adaptive reactions that help us to adjust to changing conditions. Absolute prevention replaces the concept of the cure.

Thus, in the realm of utopia, human beings will have perfected impregnable defenses against any threats to their health. But will that perfection suffice to let us lead lives without disease? Before I answer, let me ask more questions. What happens if humankind abuses its control of nature? What becomes of humans if they can control nature but cannot cope with conditions of their own making? In either event there would be a resurgence of disease.

Indiscriminate dominance over nature will cause shifts in the population of plants and animals. These changes may at first be insignificant, knowingly initiated or tolerated by humankind, but they soon would proliferate through chain reactions that are beyond human control. These profound shifts must deprive humans of vital needs. They will starve, thirst, freeze, or overheat. They may be smothered by swarms of insects after eradicating the insect-eating animals. Any one of these catastrophic events means human suffering, damage to tissues or organs, and therefore disease.

Physical suffering of human origin may assume huge proportions and is not subject to the healing or preventive medical facilities that are normally available. Modern warfare exposes entire nations to bomb blasts, burns, toxic gases, and radiation sickness. Even in times devoid of any open warfare, there are victims of political, racial, or ethnic persecution who, as inmates of prison camps, lose their health because of bad conditions and inhumane treatment.

Disease of an individual body is not much different from disease of a nation. Either one may lead to the other. Sickness of the mind, affecting just one person in power, can plunge the world into darkness, and political violence will kill its victims or destroy their health. At the root of any disease is the loss of harmony, the failing linkage between a biological unit and the world around it.

The challenge to the human species goes far beyond a mandate for perfect methods of disease prevention. Designing new techniques is as creative an activity as the formulation of a new way of government. The mind is at its best when it can be creative, busily replacing the old with the new. John Dewey wrote, "Every important satisfaction of an old want creates a new one; and this new one has to enter upon an experimental adventure to find its satisfaction."[3]

But the new requires scrutiny, analysis, and possibly rejection, sober functions of the mind that are less satisfying than creation. New cures fall into the category of creations. They are inventions or discoveries, and perfecting them is exciting and thrilling, for it fulfills the human need to fashion the new. A breakthrough in the field of prevention is hailed as a creative accomplishment only when it represents a positive method, such as a new vaccine or a drug that confers immunity against certain diseases. Noncreative measures that advocate avoidance, adjustment, or compensation are less spectacular and therefore apt to be neglected.

Nevertheless, these lackluster efforts involving dry and tedious work are vital if we want to minimize disease instead of having to repair the damage that disease inflicts. The record of the past assures us that we are capable of avoiding disease consciously. Vaccination against smallpox and prevention of scurvy with citrus juice date back to the eighteenth century. Standing between the past and the future, contemporary humans have inherited the fruit of genius and labor from centuries gone by, but we have also adopted the conviction that disease, if banished, often appears in the form of another evil and that we are destined to live with some burden regardless of our efforts.

Judging from the territory that has been conquered in a few centuries, our outlook might be brighter than most of us think. If the past and the future could speak to each other, their dialogue would be cause for hope.

> FIRST VOICE: I am the voice of the past and I speak with authority, for I state humankind's experience through the centuries. Humans possess all the physical equipment that keeps the animals alive, makes them adjust to their environment, and heals their wounds if they fail in this adjustment. But humans surpass all other creatures by their ability to act on their own, independent of natural instincts. Through the ages humans have had to satisfy their urge to find new ways of providing food, shelter, and health. It has brought them countless blessings, but in their wake came as many sorrows. For any innovation has its side effects that the innovator does not see. Nature maintains a delicate balance that no being can upset with impunity. While humankind designs brilliant devices for better living, new hazards are incurred. One burden is simply swapped for another, leaving the total load unchanged.

> SECOND VOICE: I am the spirit of the future, and I exceed the past in authority, for the centuries yet to come will use the experience of those gone by. The human mind is more than a one-track machine. True, it has an incessant need to create, but it can also remember and anticipate. In its memory bank are stored the undesirable complications that accompany the inventions of the past. Slowly but surely, humans are becoming more circumspect in their fight against disease. A new cure or a new preventive tech-

nique will be carefully observed for its side effects before it is released to the public.

FIRST VOICE: Your argument may be sound if you consider only the health industry. But disease, and I mean *physical* disease, is not confined to medical matters. Technical advances and changes of the environment can cause disease. The discoveries of radioactivity and nuclear fission or fusion are responsible for physical conditions occupying many pages in the textbooks of pathology, and perhaps . . .

SECOND VOICE: All true, but again, scrutiny and forethought will minimize the ill effects of future technology. Engineers, chemists, and manufacturers will be guided by experience. Progress must become a docile animal, tamed and bridled by caution.

FIRST VOICE: You did not let me finish. I meant to say that perhaps the greatest peril to humankind comes from the destructive acts of humans, and I refer specifically to the *purposely* destructive acts and their consequences. The ravages of modern warfare encompass a wide spectrum of physical conditions: injuries, radiation sickness, and swelling of the lungs from war gases. These are just a few examples. A victim of atrocities, slowly dying from starvation, differs little from a patient with incurable cancer. What was it that brought the starving prisoner to this terminal illness? The restless creativity of the human mind made someone think of an innovation in the exercise of power—a new form of government promising a great future to many by dooming a few to imprisonment and death. It was this person's cherished idea. He or she labored feverishly to see it become reality, just like the inventor of a piece of machinery. And this idea, born of the need to innovate, became the cause of a fatal malady for millions. Can you now deny that disease will always be with human beings, whether they live in the next century or ten centuries from now? Do you not see the obvious implication of all this? Human beings are destined to meet a certain measure of suffering. By using their ingenuity, they defy the verdict of fate, but in doing so they create new adversities for themselves. The amount of suffering does not change.

SECOND VOICE: I am almost ready to concede. Almost, but not quite! I admit that the future cannot promise that the terrors of the past will not recur. On the contrary, they are likely to return in one form or another during the coming centuries. And I must also agree that human evils differ but little from naturally occurring disease in their devastating effect. The destructive role of humans actually extends beyond the specters of war and oppression. The disruption of the environment is just beginning to be recognized as a hazard to health. The human spirit of enterprise and reform is responsible for incursions into the domain of nature, bringing immediate benefits and causing also delayed ill effects. In the vast total of all inanimate objects and all living creatures, there exists a critical balance between each part and the whole. Slight shifts in these relations influence the physical conditions of individuals. Humankind has not yet learned to foresee what each of its remodeling projects will do to the overall structure and to the component parts. But it is precisely this realization of the need for learning that lets the future gain strength from the past and find ground for optimism. Humankind's ability to learn from experience has been sufficiently documented to convince the skeptics that it will eventually foresee the side effects of its inventions.

FIRST VOICE: Let us say that humans will at least know that any new device or method, regardless of how beneficial it may be, has unexpected drawbacks. The voice of the past is the voice of the skeptics, for the past has witnessed disaster brought on by human innovations many times in each century. Still, even the most severe skeptic need not be without hope, and it is on this subject of hope that the past must yield to the future. The human mind can be trained to avoid errors, pitfalls, and oversights while reaching for new concepts.

SECOND VOICE: The keynote of any training is a wider horizon. There are no independent biological units. No creature can function alone; each must act in concert with others and is actually a functioning part in a delicately balanced mechanism. It is the specific function of *Homo sapiens* to conceive the new and to introduce it without disturbing the balance of the biological system.

FIRST VOICE: A formidable task. Almost a contradiction in itself. How can you maintain an equilibrium of forces as numerous and vast as those to which life on earth is subject? Imagine a mathematician trying to bring order into a system with endless variations of constants that are indefinite in number. The ablest minds would need an eternity to determine which combinations of vital factors are compatible with maintained balance and which are not.

SECOND VOICE: But human genius will find a way through this jungle. Already millions of different combinations can be quickly tabulated with the help of the computer and their effects compared. There will be combinations that are known to be harmonious and others that are mismatched. Any incompatible groupings lead to disease, whether they involve atoms or highly complex organisms. Disease is a warning signal, the indicator of incompatibility. The future will see a steady reduction of disease because science can learn to distinguish between permissible and harmful variations of constants.

FIRST VOICE: You seem to give little credit to the past, when much of the fight against disease was an attempt at cure or alleviation of pain. Are you implying that in the future prevention will replace healing?

SECOND VOICE: If I were, I would speak for millennia, not centuries. Humankind's ability to anticipate and forestall would have to be perfect before the healing art becomes obsolete. The fight against pain and disability has met with brilliant success, and its benefits are immediately apparent, whereas the results of prevention are more slowly appreciated. Healing means palpable relief from suffering. Prevention is intangible. How does one value the absence of pain that has never started? Above all, disease will plague humankind in one form or another for a very long time to come; prevention will probably never succeed in wiping it out entirely. And as long as people are subject to suffering, there must be remedies that bring immediate relief.

FIRST VOICE: You are now exonerating the past and projecting its role into the future. Furthermore, you have added the justified hope that in the future humankind will live with less disease than now. This seems like a good note on which to end our debate.

SECOND VOICE: I know a better note. It is true that the future will not abolish the efforts of the past but will continue them at a greatly accelerated pace. But progress will require a new concept of disease, which must be seen as a disturbance of interaction. This concept applies to the communications between biological units and also to the relations between each unit and inanimate objects or substances. Human beings are the only creatures that can make decisions based on experience and conclusions. Their decisions determine the presence of health or disease in their own lives and in the lives of all other creatures. Humankind must first learn what options are available. It must determine next the specific effect of each option, and it must finally realize its obligation to act on all options. The humans of the future will not simply delegate the care of their health to a group of professionals but will be conscious of their own roles in shaping their health.

FIRST VOICE: The past has seen the emergence of the individual's responsibility in setting his or her own course. This self-determination requires a vast pool of knowledge before a person can select wisely and quickly from a number of options. In the future the sequence of learning–deliberating–deciding will have to be intensified many times. The response to this demand will ultimately determine whether men, women, and children get the state of health they deserve.

SECOND VOICE: Or the state of disease they deserve!

10

Living Is Necessary

Life was meant to be lived, and curiosity
must be kept alive. One must never, for
whatever reason, turn his back on life.

—Eleanor Roosevelt, *Autobiography*

When Pompei the Great was warned
by his advisers that he might endanger his life by going to sea in pirate-
infested waters, he replied, "Going to sea is necessary. Living is not necessary." The remark was calculated to serve Pompei's public image as a
courageous general who considered his life expendable for the sake of the
state.

The general's rhetoric may sound good in a Latin textbook, but it hardly reflects reality. Living *is* necessary. The urge to live and to procreate is
the dominant motive in biology. Each biological unit, be it human or
amoeba, is constantly acting to ensure its survival. A unit is actually a
biological system composed of multiple entities. Even the unicellular organisms contain a variety of components within their protoplasm and
constitute an assembly of parts, each having special functions essential to
the entire unit.

Each system depends for its sustenance on the external milieu, with
which it must be in constant communication. This contact with the out-

side is the lifeline of every creature. None can exist in a vacuum. Human beings cannot divorce themselves from this need any more than the amoeba can, although they may make ingenious arrangements for temporary independence. When humans go to the moon they carry oxygen, food, water, and heating apparatus into a milieu that would not support them without these things. They nonetheless remain dependent on the earth's atmosphere, and they die if they do not get back before their supply is depleted.

The need to live thus means for each system the need to interact smoothly with the external milieu. Failure to maintain a flawlessly synchronized and coordinated action results in a deviation from the optimal biological state. This deviation represents disease and threatens life.

All beings are engaged in competition for the life-maintaining force of the external world. The losers' deaths make space and vital matter available to new competitors. It is necessary that life continue. It is consequently necessary that those whose capacity to perform vital functions is impaired must yield their places to others. Disease is the signal of impaired function, not its cause. Disease exists when, for example, the body cannot readily exchange carbon dioxide for oxygen, maintain its fluid balance, or replace lost proteins and minerals. Disease presages the end of the biological system, just as a lame gait marks the wounded deer for the wolves' assault. A pragmatic mechanism designed to ensure survival of the fittest, to permit life only at its optimal level? Perhaps. If this concept were true, then the meaning of "living is necessary" would amount to a final, chilling truth: there must be uninterrupted existence of biological units that are in total harmony with their external setting. Those that fail to keep pace are expendable.

This bleak view of life, although based on believable conclusions, is nevertheless incompatible with human nature. The necessity of life means to each person that his or her life is necessary, not just the biologically perfect life. Humans, like other animals, have a natural attachment to life and, beyond that, a conscious will to escape death as long as possible. Any sentiment that is directed against life is abnormal, motivated rarely by noble sacrifice, more often by intolerable suffering, and commonly by mental derangement.

The causes of suicide have been analyzed by philosophers, theologians, and medical specialists. Judgment of it ranges widely from sin and criminal offense to justifiable escape. Freud interpreted the death wish as a form of aggression that may turn on a loved person or on the self. Ernest

Jones, Freud's biographer, quotes from his writings: "Perhaps no one can find the psychical energy to kill himself unless in the first place he is thereby killing at the same time someone with whom he has identified himself, and is directing against himself a death wish which had previously been directed against the other person."[1]

Great thinkers have occasionally considered the thought of self-destruction acceptable or even desirable. Friedrich Nietzsche declared, "The thought of suicide is a powerful comfort; it helps one through many a dreadful night."[2]

Fanaticism and mass suggestion may lead to epidemics such as the mass suicide in Guyana in 1978. Despair or illness may move even a great mind toward a longing for death. In a letter to his father in 1787, Wolfgang Amadeus Mozart wrote, "Since death, when we come to consider it, is seen to be the true goal of our life, I have made acquaintance during these last few years with this best and truest friend of mankind, so that his image not only no longer has any terrors for me, but suggests, on the contrary, much that is reassuring and consoling!"[3]

Nevertheless, preoccupation with death and acts or thoughts of self-destruction are negligible compared to the human will to live. Even the despair of old age creates only a temporary readiness to die that in the end yields to the renewed yearning for life:

> Vainly do old men pray for death
> Regretting their age
> And the long span of life.
> If death draws near,
> None wants to die,
> And age is no more a burden to him.[4]

If we regard life as desirable and necessary, we should have a clear concept of its antagonist. The idea of death itself is too vague to serve as an image of antilife. How can one fight something that is not only inevitable but also unknowable—a concept characterized by the absence of everything that the mind associates with existence?

Being unable to wrestle with death, we turn to a compromise. We can fight disease and thereby protect life. Disease is antilife. It is allied with death, and we have come to regard it as an alien force. Disease is an invader and a destroyer. To deal with it we need trained experts who are dedicated to the preservation of life, much as we must have an army to keep enemies from our land.

It seems strange that disease, death's ally, is actually a life process. We are in constant competition with other creatures and therefore exposed to friction, injury, or extinction. Living is not an automatic, predictable occurrence but depends on interactions subject to change every second. To say that living is necessary means that effort, competition, and hazard are necessary.

Disease is not an intruder in this drama of motion and collision. It is in fact not an active participant but a condition reflecting a fault in the highly complex performance. If a thorn penetrates the sole of my foot, there is pain that draws my attention to the site of the injury. I will examine my foot and extract the thorn. The pain was an alarm signal. Without it, the thorn might have penetrated farther, causing serious disruption of tissues with blood loss and possible infection.

Like the pain of injury, disease is an alarm signal. Somewhere there is a faulty connection, an imbalance between the reactions inside the body and the conditions on its outside. It is the failure of interaction that destroys life, while the disease, with all its pain and discomfort, is only the effect that is most noticeable to us.

If we want to protect life, we must correct or prevent the imbalance that lies at the root of disease. Humans and other animals have automatic means of correction, such as elevation of body temperature and mobilization of white blood cells to combat infection. The bleeding animal may drink water to counteract the loss of fluid. This is a built-in mechanism, which is all that the animal has for protection. Humans will resort to the human-made protection, perhaps controlling the bleeding with sutures and combating blood loss with transfusions. Nonetheless, such procedures are often still primitive. Many of our methods are not designed to keep an even biological balance but deal with the symptoms after the loss of balance has become noticeable. This means that there must first be malfunction that brings disease and physical destruction.

Repair is not always possible, but this does not detract from the achievements of medical science, since future progress will overcome many of its present limitations. More important, prevention is assuming an increasingly greater role and, if successful, will make attempts at repair obsolete.

The progress of medicine is often viewed within the framework of only the last 150 years. Compared to modern methods, the achievements of medical science before 1850 are regarded as insignificant. On closer analysis, however, this attitude seems unfounded and unfair. Medicine as we know it today rests on foundations that were laid by scientists of many centuries. Antibiotics, vaccines, or bypass operations are unthinkable without mathematics, physics, and chemistry. Recent generations are reaping more tangible benefits from what has been achieved, but they cannot justly claim all the credit for their successes.

We should view progress in medicine as a gradual, steady advance along a road that has no end. Human life expectancy in the United States attained a record high of 73.2 years in 1977, and the upward trend has continued since then. The health industry has for the most part succeeded in alleviating pain and preserving life.

Humans compete with other beings for limited supplies of oxygen, light, warmth, water, and food. Our minds give us a tremendous advantage over other forms of life, but our great discoveries and inventions often bring with them new hazards. The gasoline engine causes smog and fatal accidents. The chemical industry makes toxic fumes. Atomic energy is linked to radiation sickness and birth defects, and by fighting disease with ingenious drugs, we have created new disorders known as the iatrogenic diseases. It seems that whenever we try to improve on nature, we must expect to pay a price.

Disease is a state of failure, a painful signal warning us that all is not well. Life is in jeopardy because the organism is not perfectly attuned to its external state. Through medical science we can relieve the symptoms and prolong life, but although the alarm is silenced, the basic imbalance often persists. Many of the older survivors are in suboptimal physical condition, and their further maintenance places an increasing burden on society.

What do these drawbacks mean as we watch the death rate decline and the average length of life rise each year? They mean little at present. We must protect life, except in certain terminal conditions when the last vital spark would die without the support of machines. There can be no question about the kind of population we are building. "Living is necessary" applies to everyone, not just the physically fit.

When we project our thoughts into the future, we realize that humankind could come to harm by the trend toward an ever-larger number of people who are not equal to the demands of life. The species might become an inferior competitor, surviving temporarily by clever devices without being properly attuned to the medium around it.

If we detect where we are going wrong, we might gradually succeed in living longer without resorting to artifice. We could remain in a competitive position as long as we are able to interact smoothly with our surroundings. Disease, the indicator of imbalance, would be minimized, and disease fighting would take second place to disease prevention.

This preventive approach to the health problem lacks much of the excitement and glory that surround research into the cures of disease. The discovery of a vaccine against a dread disease, for instance, may be dramatic and receive the popular recognition that it deserves. The poliomyelitis vaccine is an example of striking progress that was verified and acclaimed almost immediately after it was announced. More often, however, the use of a new vaccine is controversial, its merits becoming apparent slowly and in piecemeal fashion.

Until recently the public has been unimpressed by preventive measures that did not involve vaccines or drugs and lacked luster if compared to the discovery of insulin or penicillin. It is difficult to conceive of warnings against smoking or against exposure to asbestos as great advances in medicine, even if compliance with these warnings might prevent thousands of deaths each year. Research programs aimed at significant factors of environment and life-style are beginning to receive increasing recognition, however. The results of the American Cancer Prevention Study of 1959–79 and of the Framingham study have firmly established the need for large-scale prospective projects. They hold the promise of insight into our relationship to the environment. As we discover new risk factors, we will learn to avoid them by adjusting our habits and selecting our food in accordance with the new knowledge. Disease will occur less frequently and decrease in severity as humankind learns more and more about avoidable risks.

The basic pattern of prevention is already discernible, and the principal avenues leading to this goal have been opened. Slowly, through research and ingenuity, we may learn to avoid disease by dodging, resistance, and early suppression. We dodge disease when we eliminate its main causes through control of diet and habits. We resist it by stimulating our defenses through vaccination. We suppress disease after detecting it in its subclinical stage through screening programs.

When enough of these methods have been perfected, the increased life expectancy will become meaningful, because the disabilities of old age will be minimized. Death comes when the balance is at last gone, after many episodes of subclinical disease have gradually impaired the body's vital systems. This new kind of longevity may be slow in coming, yet we are even now moving toward it. Each of us wants to live as long as life is enjoyable and has some quality. The length and kind of life depend on the ability of the organism to relate harmoniously to the medium within which it exists. By furthering this harmony we can have a longer life and make old age more desirable.

What kind of use will there be for the multitudes of the future? Where will they live and what will they eat? These questions are unanswerable now, but we expect that answers will be found. Pompei, it seems, was wrong. It *is* necessary to live! Going to sea, tunneling into the earth, and rocketing through space will receive their due share of attention from us as long as we retain our physical fitness.

We have the gift of thought, a tool with which we can alter the course of events. We improve our living conditions by putting technical inventions to work. Any new advance may eliminate some adverse effects of the environment but may open the door to others. Even if we wish to preserve animal life, we are reducing it steadily by industrial and residential expansion. We regard these as essential, although we are hurting ourselves by inflicting damage on the environment. Pollution of air, water, and soil has toxic effects, and many pollutants have been identified as carcinogens. Displacement or eradication of wildlife interferes with the control of insects, some of which are carriers of infectious diseases.

Despite the known hazards, we will continue to tamper with the living and inanimate world around us. If we refrain from doing so, we will lose the comforts of our daily lives, such as heating, lighting, transportation, and ample choice of food. We will never stop acting on our own and exploring new avenues that we believe will lead to our own advancement. We must follow the ambitious designs born of the intricate function of our brains, just as the wolf must hunt and the beaver must build dams.

Rights and Obligations

I believe that every right implies a responsibility;
every opportunity, an obligation; every possession,
a duty.

—John D. Rockefeller

The right of every human being to receive medical care is a concept that few if any would dispute. But this is an abstract idea unless it is implemented by concrete expressions. If we were to speak first of obligations, we might find it easier to understand rights. Society has an obligation to care for its sick. This statement defies any challenge or discretion, for the thought that suffering should be ignored is obscene and absurd. It is obscene because it violates accepted laws of decency; it is absurd because if put into effect, it would weaken and eventually destroy society.

If we accept the idea of group responsibility, it follows that each member of the group has an obligation. We consider the health of the group important; therefore, each of us must participate in this effort. The duty is twofold. First, it comprises strengthening the community effort to provide health care. In addition, it demands the individual's continued effort to maintain his or her own health.

The individual's task is one that requires personal decisions on matters that are often not clear and await confirmation or rejection through long-term research. Our habits and life-styles shape our state of health, but we have authoritative guidelines for only a few facts. The rest is circumstantial evidence, and each of us must decide the bases on which to govern the conduct of his or her own life. It is our obligation to select a life-style that we consider conducive to health and to follow this plan with perseverance. When we recognize our responsibilities and live up to them, we are in a better position to speak of our right to health care.

Preventing or overcoming disease means utilizing natural mechanisms that go into action when they are needed. They occur automatically in animals and human beings. We have enforced the natural defenses with measures of our own design. We avoid yellow fever by eradicating the mosquito that carries the virus. We prevent smallpox by stimulating the production of antibodies through vaccination. We fight bacteria with extracts from molds, and we repair clogged arteries, replacing them with veins or synthetic products.

Speculating about the future often amounts only to idle thoughts, but thinking of what is to come exceeds mere conjecture if it is based on past experience. The record of achievements in medicine suggests a brilliant future. Remedies are already available for many of the most dreaded infections. It is important to recall the scourges of a generation or so ago, such as diphtheria, meningitis, tetanus, poliomyelitis, and endocarditis. Today we take prevention or cure of these for granted. At the same time, surgery and internal medicine are making new inroads against heart disease. Even many forms of cancer are now curable. Prevention, perhaps the most important of all health measures, has taken giant strides with vaccinations, sanitary measures, prenatal care, and the reduction of infant mortality.

Idle thoughts? Hardly. We have a right to anticipate future developments as long as they are reasonable projections that we can back up with facts. Making these conclusions is more than license; it is an obligation. Realizing the importance of the human-made phase in the fight against disease eliminates any excuse for a passive attitude. We get what we deserve. Our daily choices affect our own welfare and that of future generations. We are responsible.

During the second half of the twentieth century this awareness of our collective responsibility has brought about vast changes that affect both the providers of health care and its recipients. In Europe many physicians in the early decades of this century displayed an air of superiority toward their patients by continuing traditions of past centuries. Assuming that their patients were generally uneducated and not too knowledgeable about medicine, physicians liked to confer with each other in Latin at the bedside. Patients received brief instructions without much explanation and with little room for choice. In the teaching hospitals sick men, women, or children were commonly shown to large groups of students with little regard for the patients' feelings or rights to privacy.

Within the health profession the authority of the doctors was generally absolute. They disliked any criticism or request for consultation by their colleagues. The role of the nurses resembled that of servants, regardless of their training and experience. The hospitals observed a discipline approaching that of schools and sometimes the military. Strict regulations were enforced, and treatments prescribed by the physicians were seldom subject to argument. The doctrine of informed consent may have been taught to students in law schools, but it had not yet entered the doctor-patient relationship.

Today's improved conditions stem mainly from emphasis on the dignity of the individual, human rights, and the demands of a more knowledgeable public, but there are other ingredients to the changed recipe. The rapid advances in all fields of medicine have made doctors realize their need for specialists, consultants, and postgraduate education. They must scrutinize all phases of their practice in each case, for legal decisions have made them vulnerable to litigation on causes that a plaintiff's lawyer would not have pursued a few decades earlier.

The ranks of the medical professionals are no longer limited to physicians but now include also registered nurses, medical laboratory technologists, and pharmacists, as well as X-ray technicians and other qualified technical specialists. All these professionals are bound by their codes of ethics. They are expected to voice objections should any doctor's orders conflict with the firmly established rules of each individual specialty.

Hospitals have become complex institutions with staffs of trained administrators. These administrators are in charge of finances, planning, buying, quality control, employment, public relations, and many other functions, particularly the observance of all the involved and frequently changing government regulations.

The patient is the central figure in the vast health industry. His or her welfare is the ultimate goal of the combined efforts that the providers make day and night. The planning, new methods, and rules are designed to guarantee the greatest comfort and the best physical condition possible to the men, women, and children who are their beneficiaries. While gaining new privileges, however, the recipients of health care have also acquired obligations that hardly would have been considered during the early decades of this century. The industry's performance depends to a great extent on the public's cooperation. To minimize the impact of disease, it is no longer enough to seek professional advice, for the doctors may offer several options rather than one firm recommendation.

The abundance of new research and the early release of data often make more than one method appear promising. This is especially true in the realm of prevention. For example, the preventive value of aspirin taken regularly seems fairly well established for victims of a previous heart attack,[1] but will it keep others from having their first attack, and how does this method affect the occurrence of stroke? Should persons with a moderately high level of cholesterol take medication or rely on diet and exercise? Do minor elevations of blood pressure necessitate treatment with drugs? Should all pigmented moles be excised? In time, reliable answers will be found to many of these questions.

New medical or surgical methods need not reveal their undesirable effects for long periods of time. In years past babies were sometimes treated with X rays because their thymus glands seemed to be enlarged, and this condition was regarded as a potential cause of sudden death in infants. When the children who had been so treated became teenagers or young adults, they had a relatively high incidence of cancer of the thyroid.[2] The thyroid and thymus glands are located near each other, so both would have received the radiation that occasionally had a delayed carcinogenic effect on the thyroid. The entire theory of the enlarged thymus, moreover, has since been disproved.

Making choices is one of the obligations of those who benefit from the progress of medicine. They must not only decide on a suitable life-style but have sufficient discipline to follow its demands. An important decision is the choice of a physician, which requires information based on inquiries, the experience of other patients, and possibly a preliminary discussion with the prospective doctor. Obtaining a second opinion about a recommended course of treatment is often not merely a privilege but also a responsibility that the patient owes to him- or herself.

Much of the individual person's obligation relates to the financing of health care. The cost of medical services is escalating at an unbelievable rate.[3] In 1989 medical services represented about 11.5 percent of the U.S. gross national product, whereas the corresponding figure was about 3.5

percent twenty-five years earlier.[4] To be prepared for all medical expenses, the average person must make an adequate budgetary allowance and obtain significant insurance coverage. In the light of the frequent changes in the rates and regulations, this means businesslike decisions based on periodic reviews of insurance plans and personal finances.

We must furnish access to high-level care not only for ourselves but also for those who cannot pay for themselves. Some of the privileged are improving the health of the poor through voluntary contributions, whereas others participate only by paying their taxes, which allows the government to finance insurance plans.

The care that individuals receive regardless of their own means varies in type and degree from one country to another, ranging from little free care to completely socialized medicine. If one looks at the entire world population, the task of reducing the suffering from disease still seems immense. The World Health Organization reported in 1989 that in the poor countries of Africa, Asia, and South America, health expenditures per person still average only a small fraction of the comparable figure in the United States, Canada, Japan, and western Europe. Furthermore, millions of unvaccinated children in the poor countries die annually from preventable diseases, including poliomyelitis, tetanus, measles, diphtheria, and whooping cough. Many other ailments are fatal to millions of children who could have been be cured if resources were available. This category includes diarrheal diseases, pneumonia, and tuberculosis.

In spite of the somber tone these figures cast, there is cause for hope. Human life expectancy has been raised more than ten years in the developing countries over the last forty years. Immunization in these countries has increased from 5 percent to 60 percent in ten years. The last case of smallpox was reported in 1979, and the virtual eradication of this disease has saved an estimated 20,000 lives worldwide.

If we project the achievements of health care into the distant future, we are entitled to expect many present diseases to disappear, whereas others may emerge. Some of these will be iatrogenic conditions stemming from complications of medical treatment.[5] More important is our constantly growing exposure to harmful agents—radiation, chemical substances, noise, psychological stress, and many others that can disrupt the smooth functioning of our bodies. Of greatest concern at this time is the spread of the AIDS epidemic.

Living in a crowded community with other creatures, we are in constant competition with animals, microbes, and viruses. Our competitors often have an advantage over us. They may adapt better to extreme temperatures, excel in physical strength, or be indifferent to drying. Some infiltrate our tissues without warning. Invariably, however, our inventive minds find substitutes or remedies for the shortcomings of our bodies. We can see the bacteria and viruses through ingeniously designed microscopes, tame the largest animal, stand on the bottom of the sea, and walk on the surface of the moon. Clearly, we are superior in competing not only for food, water, and oxygen but also for health.

We try to use our superiority to prevent or combat the effects of the natural scourges, such as famines, floods, or storms. In this effort we are aided by rational explanations of each disaster. The scourge that we call disease so far has yielded only some of its secrets. We know that it is not simply a hostile force attacking us from outside. We think of it as a wide spectrum of disturbances affecting our bodies or our minds and causing suffering in one form or another. This simple definition, however, does not help us to understand our role in the complex nature of disease.

If we see each organism as a fraction of all living matter, we realize that each must interact with the whole and that undisturbed life requires constant adjustment to changes occurring outside the organism. Disease in any form indicates that the process of adjustment is inadequate. It is our responsibility to forestall or minimize any failures of adjustment. This obligation goes far beyond making periodic visits to the doctor's office. It requires attention to the facts of health care in its widest sense, ranging from one person's life-style to worldwide financing of disease prevention.

Many of today's convalescents would have died from their ailments had they lived fifty years ago. If there was so much progress in half a century, is it then not possible, or even probable, that at some time in the future humans will lead lives free of any painful or disabling illness? They will be protected by their natural defense mechanisms combined with all the curative and preventive measures amassed through many centuries by the labor of uncounted men and women. Disease will not have disappeared, but death will come after a considerably longer life and will be due to the cumulative effect of many subclinical episodes of disease that caused no significant suffering.

The people of the future may think of us, the ancient people, as having lived in unbelievable ignorance. They nevertheless might give us some credit and say that we were dimly aware of our responsibility to progress and had laid the groundwork for the fight against disease.

As some of the people who will be "ancient" to the people of the future, today's convalescents believe that they are living up to their responsibilities. Their deaths have been postponed through the progress of medicine, however primitive this may seem in the distant future. They enjoy feelings of renewed strength and the comfort of easy breathing and of moving about without distress. The sunlight filtering through the foliage no longer hurts their eyes. It makes them think of life rebounding, the bright flame of life that burns on and on.

The human mind is not equipped to get a clear image of the meaning of eternity. Time without end is but a nebulous void. But one can imagine the lifespan of a generation over and over again, a thousand times and beyond. Will life on earth continue that long? Each of us, at some time, is tempted to agree with the cynics who declare that the insane acts of humankind will surely succeed in destroying all life on the planet. Our thoughts, however, soon find their way out of this valley of doom.

To think of life as something destined to end violates a feeling that is deeply ingrained in human nature. We must accept the death of the individual plant, animal, or human being, but anticipating the end of all life is absurd—a contrived view that is contrary to all natural concepts. How can it make sense to believe that all vital activity, with its endless variations of movement, color, and sound, exists only to be eventually frozen in motionless silence?

Belief in impending doom, personal or universal, goes against the evidence provided by nature that everywhere bespeaks survival. There is greening after the drought and new movement after the wintry sleep. Each creature strives for resurgence of its strength after disease has struck. Humans, above all other creatures, have the power to fight the ravages of disease. This fight is the task of all, for all of us must help to sustain the flame of life for ourselves, our contemporaries, and the generations to come.

Notes

Chapter 1: Into the Void

1. Quoted in L. Renou, *Hinduism* (New York: George Brazilier, 1962), 73.

Chapter 2: The Unit and the Whole

1. R. Virchow, "Cellular Pathology," in *Disease, Life and Man: Selected Essays by Rudolf Virchow,* trans. and with an introduction by Leland J. Rather (Stanford: University of California Press, 1958), 243.

2. C. Bernard, *Lectures on the Phenomena of Life, Common to Animals and Plants,* trans. Hebbel E. Hoff, Roger Guillemin, and Lucienne Guillemin (Springfield, Ill.: Charles C. Thomas, 1974), 1:83–84.

3. W. B. Cannon, *The Wisdom of the Body* (New York: Norton, 1963).

4. Z. Harsanyi and R. Hutton, *Genetic Prophecy: Beyond the Double Helix* (New York: Rawson, Wade, 1981), 40.

5. H. Selye, *The Stress of Life* (New York: McGraw-Hill, 1956).

6. Ibid., 118.

7. Ibid., 127

8. F. M. Burnet, "The New Approach to Immunology," *New England Journal of Medicine* 264 (1961): 24–34.

9. H. Spencer, "First Principles," in *The Age of Ideology,* ed. H. D. Aiken, 161–82 (New York: New American Library, 1956), 180, 182.

Chapter 3: The Risks of Living

1. P. Pott, *Chirurgical Observations Relative to the Cataract, the Polypus of the Nose, the Cancer of the Scrotum, the Different Kinds of the Ruptures and the Mortification of the Toe and Fat* (London: Hawes, Clark and Collins, 1775);

reprinted in *First International Conference on the Biology of Cutaneous Cancer,* 7–13, National Cancer Institute Monograph no. 10 (Philadelphia: National Cancer Institute, 1962), 12.

2. K. Yamagiwa and K. Ichikawa, "Experimental Study of the Pathogenesis of Carcinoma," *Journal of Cancer Research* 3 (1918): 1–29.

3. J. W. Cook and E. L. Kennaway, "Chemical Compounds as Carcinogenic Agents," *American Journal of Cancer* 33 (1938): 50–97.

4. I. J. Selikoff, E. C. Hammond, and J. Churg, "Asbestos Exposure, Smoking and Neoplasia," *Journal of the American Medical Association* 204 (1968): 106–12.

5. F. X. Mahoney, "Saccharin's Link to Human Cancer Questioned," *Journal of the National Cancer Institute* 84 (1992): 665.

6. R. O. Eggeberg et al., "Report to the Secretary of HEW from the Medical Advisory Group on Cyclamates," *Journal of the American Medical Association* 211 (1970): 1358–61.

7. R. W. Tennant and B. G. Margolin, "Prediction of Chemical Carcinogenity in Rodents from *In Vitro* Genetic Toxicity Assays," *Science* 236 (1987): 1933–41.

8. U. Saffiotti, "The Laboratory Approach to the Identification of Environmental Carcinogens," in *Proceedings of the Ninth Canadian Cancer Research Conference,* ed. P. G. Scholefield, 23–36 (Toronto: University of Toronto Press, 1971).

9. J. B. Heinrich, "The Postmenopausal Estrogen/Breast Cancer Controversy," *Journal of the American Medical Association* 260 (1992): 1900–1901.

10. J. E. Craighead, "Environmental Pathology," *Archives of Pathology and Laboratory Medicine* 103 (1979): 325–26.

11. P. G. Shields and C. C. Harris, "Environmental Causes of Cancer," *Medical Clinics of North America* 79 (1990): 263–77.

12. A. Ochsner and M. DeBakey, "Carcinoma of the Lung," *Archives of Surgery* 42 (1941): 209–58.

13. *American Cancer Society Cancer Prevention Study, 1959–1979: A Report on 20 Years of Progress* (Atlanta: American Cancer Society, 1979), 1.

14. J. E. Enstrom, "Cancer Mortality among Mormons," *Cancer* 42 (1978): 1943–51.

15. J. Pruett et al., "A Multivariate Analysis of Risk of Coronary Heart Disease in Framingham," *Journal of Chronic Diseases* 20 (1967): 511–24.

16. E. Marshall, "A Is for Apple, Alar and . . . Alarmists?" *Science* 254 (1991): 20–22.

17. G. S. Patton III, "Letter to Cadet George S. Patton IV, June 6, 1944," in *Bartlett's Familiar Quotations,* 15th ed., ed. J. Barlett (Boston: Little, Brown, 1980), 791.

Chapter 4: The Causal Connection

1. J. S. Haldane, *Mechanism, Life and Personality* (London: Griffin, 1921), 61.

2. W. Durant, *The Pleasures of Philosophy* (New York: Simon and Schuster/Touchstone, 1953), 71.

3. D. P. Burkitt et al., "Effect of Dietary Fiber on Stools and Transit Time and Its Role in the Causation of Disease," *Lancet* 1 (1972): 1408–11.

4. C. R. Scriver and C. L. Clow, "Phenylketonuria: Epitome of Human Biochemical Genetics," *New England Journal of Medicine* 303 (1980): 1336–42.

5. See also J. M. McGinnis and W. H. Foege, "Actual Causes of Death in the United States," *Journal of the American Medical Association* 270 (1993): 2207–12.

6. L. Aschoff, *Lectures on Pathology* (New York: Paul B. Hoeber, 1924), 365.

7. S. A. Grover et al., "Benefits of Treating Hyperlipidemia to Prevent Coronary Heart Disease," *Journal of the American Medical Association* 267 (1992): 816–22; see also notes 6 and 8 for this chapter.

8. D. Steinberg, "Underlying Mechanism in Atherosclerosis," *Journal of Pathology* 133 (1981): 75–87.

9. P. Rous, "A Sarcoma of the Fowl, Transmissable by an Agent Separable from Tumor Cells," *Journal of Experimental Medicine* 13 (1911): 397–411.

10. C. S. Babkin et al., "Incidence of Lymphomas and Other Cancers in HIV-infected and HIV-uninfected Patients with Hemophilia," *Journal of the American Medical Association* 267 (1992): 1090–94.

11. G. J. Nuovo and B. M. Pedemonte, "Human Papillomavirus. Types and Recurrent Cervical Warts," *Journal of the American Medical Association* 263 (1990): 1223–26.

12. R. A. Weinberg, "Oncogenes and Tumor Suppressor Genes," *CA: A Cancer Journal for Clinicians* 44 (1994): 160–70.

Chapter 5: From Beginning to End

1. Hippocrates, *Hippocratic Writings,* ed. G. E. R. Lloyd; trans. J. Chadwick and W. N. Mann (New York: Pelican, 1978), 321.

2. G. Mendel, "Experiments in Plant-Hybridization," in *The World of Mathematics,* ed. J. R. Newman (New York: Simon and Schuster, 1956), 2:947.

3. H. J. Muller, "Artificial Transmutation of the Gene," *Science* 66 (1927): 84–87.

4. A. T. Hertig and J. Rock, "A Series of Potentially Abortive Ova Recovered from Fertile Women prior to the First Missed Menstrual Period," *American Journal of Obstetrics and Gynecology* 58 (1949): 968–93.

5. H. D. McConnell and D. H. Carr, "Recent Advances in the Cytogenetic Study of Human Spontaneous Abortion," *Obstetrics and Gynecology* 45 (1975): 547–52.

6. M. A. Stenchever, K. J. Parks, et al., "Cytogenetics of Habitual Abortion and Other Reproductive Wastage," *American Journal of Obstetrics and Gynecology* 127 (1977): 143–50.

7. M. T. Mennuti, "Prenatal Diagnosis—Advances Bring New Challenges" *New England Journal of Medicine* 320 (1989): 661–63.

8. J. D. Watson, F. H. C. Crick, M. H. S. Wilkins, et al., "Molecular Structure of Nucleic Acids: A Structure for Deoxyribonucleic Acid," *Nature* 171 (1953): 737–38

9. J. D. Watson, *Molecular Biology of the Gene,* 2d ed. (New York: W. A. Benjamin, 1970), 28, 29.

10. A. E. Garrod, "The Incidence of Alkaptonuria: A Study in Chemical Individuality," *Lancet* 2 (1902): 1616–20.

11. L. Pauling et al., "Sickle Cell Anemia. A Molecular Disease," *Science* 110 (1949): 543–48.

12. F. Jacob, *The Logic of Life: A History of Heredity,* trans. Betty E. Spillmann (New York: Pantheon, 1973), 1.

13. L. Fishbein, "Environmental Sources of Chemical Mutagens," in *Advances in Modern Toxicology,* ed. W. G. Flanum and M. A. Hehlman (Washington, D.C.: Hemisphere, 1978), 5:175–348.

14. J. Kline, Z. Stein, M. Susser, *Conception to Birth: Epidemiology of Prenatal Development* (New York: Oxford University Press, 1989).

15. T. J. Lawley et al., "Fetal and Maternal Risk Factors in *Herpes Gestationis,*" *Archives of Dermatology* 114 (1978): 552–55.

16. A. L. Herbst, H. Ulfelder, and D. C. Poskanzer, "Adeno-Carcinoma of the Vagina. Association of Maternal Stilbesterol Therapy with Tumor Appearance in Young Women," *New England Journal of Medicine* 248 (1971): 878–81.

17. S. Nishigaki and M. Harada, "Methylmercury and Silenium in Umbilical Cords of Inhabitants of the Minimata Area," *Nature* 258 (1975): 324–25.

18. R. T. Lie, A. J. Wilcox, and R. A. Skjaerven, "Population-based Study of the Risk of Recurrence of Birth Defects," *New England Journal of Medicine* 331 (1994): 1–4.

19. P. M. Farrell and R. D. Zachman, "Pulmonary Surfactant and the Respiratory Distress Syndrome," in *Fetal and Maternal Medicine,* ed. E. J. Quilligan and N. Kretchmer (New York: Wiley, 1980), 230.

20. J. Y. Wei, "Age and the Cardiovascular System," *New England Journal of Medicine* 327 (1992): 1735–39.

21. R. L. Walford, "The Clinical Promise of Diet Restriction," *Geriatrics* 45 (1990): 81–87.

Chapter 6: Anatomy of Disease

1. G. B. Morgagni, *De Sedibus et Causis Morborum per Anatomen Indagatis,* trans. Benjamin Alexander (New York: Hafner, 1950).

2. G. N. Papanicolaou, "Cytologic Diagnosis of Uterine Cancer by Examination of Vaginal and Uterine Secretions," *American Journal of Clinical Pathology* 19 (1949): 301.

3. C. Mettlin and C. D. Smart, "Breast Cancer Detection Guidelines for Women Aged 40–49 Years: Rationale for the American Cancer Society Reaffirmation of Recommendations," *CA: A Cancer Journal for Clinicians* 44 (1994): 248–355.

4. D. E. Henson, "Revisiting the Autopsy," *Archives of Pathology and Laboratory Medicine* 14 (1990): 127–28.

5. A. Vesalius, *De Humani Corporis Fabrica,* trans. J. B. de C. M. Saunders and C. D. O'Malley (Cleveland: World, 1950).

6. W. Harvey, "Exercitatio Anatomica De Motu Cordis et Sanguinis," in *Encyclopedia of Medical History,* ed. R. E. McGrew (New York: McGraw-Hill, 1985), 65.

7. *World Health Organization: Semi-Annual Report* (World Health Organization, 1944).

8. R. C. Gallo et al., "Frequent Detection and Isolation of Cytopathic Retroviruses from Patients with AIDS and at Risk for AIDS," *Science* 224 (1984): 500.

9. J. S. Coon et al., "Interlaboratory Variation in DNA Flow Cytometry," *Journal of Pathology and Laboratory Medicine* 118 (1994): 681–85.

10. A. A. Sandberg, "Cancer Cytogenetics for Clinicians," *CA: A Cancer Journal for Clinicians* 44 (1994): 136.

11. W. W. McLendon, "Pathologists in the 1990s and in the 21st Century," *Archives of Pathology and Laboratory Medicine* 116 (1992): 563–65.

Chapter 7: Prevention

1. G. N. Papanicolaou, "Cytologic Diagnosis of Uterine Cancer by Examination of Vaginal and Uterine Secretions," *American Journal of Clinical Pathology* 19 (1949): 301.

2. T. Mann, *The Magic Mountain,* trans. H. T. Lowe-Porter (New York: Vintage, 1969), 719.

3. Ibid., 359

4. S. A. Waksman, *The Conquest of Tuberculosis* (Berkeley: University of California Press, 1964), 117.

5. Mann, *Magic Mountain,* 285.

6. B. R. Edlin et al., "An Outbreak of Multidrug-resistant Tuberculosis

among Hospitalized Patients with Acquired Immunodeficiency Syndrome," *New England Journal of Medicine* 326 (1992): 1514.

7. E. C. Faust, P. F. Russell, and R. C. Jung, *Craig and Faust's Clinical Parasitology,* 8th ed., rev. (Philadelphia: Lea and Febiger, 1970), 42.

8. R. L. Martensen, "Oliver Wendell Holmes, M.D.: An Appreciation," *Journal of the American Medical Association* 272 (1994): 1249.

9. E. Jenner, "An Inquiry into the Causes and Effects of the Variolae Vaccinae, Known by the Name of the Cow-Pox," in *Great Adventures in Medicine,* ed. Samuel Rapport and Helen Wright, 166–75 (New York: Dial, 1961).

10. R. Vallery-Radot, "Louis Pasteur and the Conquest of Rabies," in *Great Adventures in Medicine,* ed. Samuel Rapport and Helen Wright, 262–76 (New York: Dial, 1961), 168.

11. J. G. Breman and I. Arita, "The Confirmation and Maintenance of Smallpox Eradication," *New England Journal of Medicine* 303 (1980): 1263–73.

12. W. Fields, personal communication.

13. J. G. Gorman, "Rh Immunoglobulin in Prevention of Hemolytic Disease of Newborn Child," *New York Journal of Medicine* 68 (1968): 1270–77.

14. N. C. Rose and M. T. Mennuti, "Maternal Serum Screening for Neural Tube Defects and Fetal Chromosome Abnormality," *Western Journal of Medicine* 159 (1993): 312–17.

15. S. Schmidt-Jensen, M. Permin, et al., "Randomised Comparison of Amniocentesis and Transabdominal and Transcervical Chorionic Villus Sampling," *Lancet* 340 (1992): 1237–44.

16. "Symposium on Medical Genetics," in *The Pediatric Clinics of North America,* ed. M. M. Kaback, vol. 25, no. 3, 395–409 (Philadelphia: Saunders, 1978).

Chapter 8: The Human Reaction

1. R. D. Cumming, *The Philosophy of Jean-Paul Sartre* (New York: Random House, 1968), 277, 280.

2. Epictetus, quoted in W. J. Oates, *The Stoic and Epicurean Philosophers* (New York: Random House, 1940), 361.

3. Marcus Aurelius, quoted in ibid., 539.

4. G. W. F. Hegel, "The Philosophy of History," *The Age of Ideology* (New York: New American Library, 1956), 89.

5. A. Schopenhauer, *The World as Will and Idea,* quoted in Will Durant, *The Story of Philosophy* (New York: Simon and Schuster, 1953), 238.

6. H. D. Thoreau, *Walden* (New York: New American Library, 1960), 65.

7. Alexander of Tralles, quoted in B. Inglis, *A History of Medicine* (Cleveland: World, 1965), 5.

8. Cited in V. R. Young and D. P. Richardson, "Nutrients, Vitamins, and Minerals in Cancer Prevention," *Cancer* 43, supplement (May 1979): 2125–36; quotation on 2128.

9. V. Herbert, "Unproven (Questionable) Dietary and Nutritional Methods in Cancer Prevention and Treatment," *Cancer* 58 (1986): 1930–41.

10. R. Gay, "Fear of Food," *American Scholar* 45 (1976): 437.

11. J. Dewey, *Human Nature and Conduct* (New York: Modern Library, 1957), 207.

12. D. Pittet et al., "Nosocomial Blood Stream Infection in Critically Ill Patients," *Journal of the American Medical Association* 271 (1994): 1598.

13. R. F. Breiman, J. C. Butler, et al., "Emergence of Drug-resistant Pneumococcal Infections in the United States," *Journal of the American Medical Association* 271 (1994): 1831–35.

14. M. S. Rosenschein et al., "The Cost Effectiveness of Therapeutic and Prophylactic Leukocyte Transfusion," *New England Journal of Medicine* 302 (1980): 1058–62.

Chapter 9: Dialogue of the Ages

1. C. Darwin, *The Origin of Species by Means of Natural Selection, or The Preservation of Favoured Races in the Struggle for Life* (New York: Avenel/Crown, 1966 [1859]).

2. Ibid., 441–42.

3. J. Dewey, *Human Nature and Conduct* (New York: Modern Library, 1957), 285.

Chapter 10: Living Is Necessary

1. E. Jones, *The Life and Work of Sigmund Freud*, 3 vols. (New York: Basic, 1957), 2:280.

2. F. W. Nietzsche, *Beyond Good and Evil*, trans. W. Kaufmann (New York: Vintage, 1966), 91.

3. W. A. Mozart, quoted in M. Davenport, *Mozart* (New York: Avon, 1979), 270–71.

4. Euripides, *Alcestis*, in *Seven Famous Greek Plays*, ed. Whitney J. Oates and Eugene O'Neill Jr., 235–85 (New York: Vintage, 1961), 267.

Chapter 11: Rights and Obligations

1. J. E. Willard, R. A. Lange, et al., "The Use of Aspirin in Ischemic Heart Disease," *New England Journal of Medicine* 327 (1992): 175–81.

2. A. B. Schneider et al., "Characteristics of 108 Thyroid Cancers Detected

by Screening in a Population with a History of Head and Neck Irradiation," *Cancer* 46 (1980): 1218–27.

3. G. D. Lundberg, "An Overview of Health System Reform," *Journal of the American Medical Association* 271 (1994): 1368.

4. M. Lerner, "Access to the American Health Care System: Consequences of Cancer Control," *CA: A Cancer Journal for Clinicians* 39 (1989): 289–95.

5. S. M. Wilcox, D. U. Himmelstein, et al., "Inappropriate Drug Prescribing for the Community-dwelling Elderly," *Journal of the American Medical Association* 272 (1994): 292–96.

Index

PETER M. MARCUSE, M.D., was educated in Europe and received his medical degree from the University of Basel, Switzerland. He is presently a clinical associate professor of pathology at Baylor College of Medicine. From 1949 until his retirement in 1989 he was affiliated with St. Joseph Hospital in Houston, Texas, as director of laboratories and pathologist-in-chief. He is the author of numerous articles on specific aspects of pathology, as well as of the textbook *Diagnostic Pathology in Gynecology and Obstetrics.*